Aspergers Syndrome

A Complete Aspergers Syndrome Cure Guide

(Get a More Extensive Learning About Asperger's and How to Manage It)

Eugene Gardner

Published By **Bella Frost**

Eugene Gardner

All Rights Reserved

Aspergers Syndrome: A Complete Aspergers Syndrome Cure Guide (Get a More Extensive Learning About Asperger's and How to Manage It)

ISBN 978-1-7772550-0-8

Legal & Disclaimer

The information contained in this book is not designed to replace or take the place of any form of medicine or professional medical advice. The information in this book has been provided for educational & entertainment purposes only.

The information contained in this book has been compiled from sources deemed reliable, and it is accurate to the best of the Author's knowledge; however, the Author cannot guarantee its accuracy and validity and cannot be held liable for any errors or omissions. Changes are periodically made to this book. You must consult your doctor or get professional medical advice before using any of the suggested remedies, techniques, or information in this book.

Table Of Contents

Chapter 1: Starting Kindergarten

2. My 4 12 months-vintage toddler goes to kindergarten in September. I truely have a four twelve month's antique little one who is stepping into Kindergarten in September. What information should he provide me regarding Asperger's? He moreover had problem in preschool because of his boredom, so he became called a bad boy. How can I help him adapt to kindergarten?

For your infant's training, it's far essential to shape a partnership. You understand your infant higher than surely anybody else as a discern Asperger's Syndrome is precise in that you understand your infant's strengths and weaknesses better than truely everyone. Your infant's instructors are specialists in supporting him to get the excellent training and characteristic a laugh doing it. You can artwork collectively to create the top notch plan on your infant's schooling. These are a few guidelines that will help you get started out:

Open conversation–

As quick as possible, time table a meeting with the college body of workers. Send the college body of employee's copies of any mental or medical reviews that provide statistics about your son's diagnosis. Talk approximately your son's preschool memories. Unbalanced applications are probably to have introduced about boredom and other troubles. Although Asperger's Syndrome does now not motive highbrow disabilities, a few educators might not recognize this. Asperger's Syndrome training is extra complex than simply enforcing a favored curriculum.

Request instructional evaluations

Medical reviews are unique from educational critiques. School

Evaluations might not continuously in form the analysis. The interest want to be at the services provided. If you aren't glad with the university's conclusions, you may request a 2d evaluation.

Request an Individualized Education Plan

A Individual Education Plan, or IEP, is a criminal file that offers the inspiration for your baby's special training. You may be part of the education team for your son and paintings with instructors and therapists for you to set up academic and treatment desires. These goals will help your son conquer boredom and distinct behavioral issues, if critical, and ensure his academic achievement.

Become an worried discern

Participation within the educational system is the simplest way to discover if your son has done his academic goals. Ask questions. Discuss your son's day at university with him. Participate in any determine training that is provided with the resource of the personnel. As a extremely good deal as you can, volunteer at his university. You can be diagnosed with the useful resource of the college workforce as a parent when they recognize you!

Education of your son is a team attempt. It's vital to installation sturdy, longlasting relationships with school team of workers. Teachers care deeply approximately their university students and want them to achieve success. Parents and instructors can paintings together to create a nice analyzing surroundings for kids with Asperger's Syndrome.

School Transition

three. My son will enter excessive university this fall after years of very terrible research in public schools. To put together for this transition, we've were given updated his IEP. But will we notify the college of the issues and expect upgrades or wait until they begin?

For teens with Asperger's Syndrome, excessive university may be a difficult enjoy. Teens with Asperger's have extra issues due to social awkwardness and maturity troubles. Thank you for being a proactive and involved parent. You have definitely taken many steps to make sure that your son's excessive faculty years are a fulfillment. These are extra thoughts about your son's situation.

The awesome transition

A cutting-edge IEP is a extraordinary region for a start. For a smooth transition into excessive college, you can want to address one-of-a-kind personal troubles. Discuss in conjunction with your son the differences amongst middle and immoderate college. He will want to do greater on an character basis. He need to learn how to take duty for his very very own picks simply so he can be geared up for maturity. Discuss non-public hygiene, organization, and social expectancies. These are regions in which Asperger's sufferers can show weakness.

New expectancies

This is your danger to offer your son a easy start. This is a current-day college, new personnel and a sparkling begin to your son. Write down what you count on from your son inside the coming one year. Make a listing of acceptable conduct in severa conditions to help your son. You are privy to his beyond struggles, so that you can bring together on them and hold in mind other situations. Assist him with organizing his existence at school and at domestic. Encourage him to participate in remedy and social abilties instructions.

Past behavioral troubles and a ultra-present day college

His everlasting college file will encompass any behavioral issues that your son can also moreover have had in the past. This statistics need to now not be hidden. It isn't always critical to mention the ones troubles. However, you ought to be open to being asked. Your son has in reality noted this trouble with you and said which you expect improvement. Don't borrow problems. They may not come! Prepare to cope with any new problems head-on with the faculty management as a group.

Enlightening the group of workers

It is critical which you set up relationships with the body of humans at your son's university. It is viable that employee's contributors do not know an entire lot approximately Asperger's Syndrome. You have to maintain a concise summary of Autism Spectrum Disorder and Asperger's Syndrome to your son's everlasting record Also, replica and offer copies to each of his instructors.

You've taken steps to assist your son transition effortlessly into a brand new segment of his existence. You can count on superb opportunities and new reviews on this new season.

Relocation

four. I'm considering moving to a ultra-modern-day domestic, if you need to additionally imply changing colleges for my Asperger's 11-twelve months antique son. Please, any advice?

Moving equals change. This is specially right for Asperger's Syndrome kids. Asperger's Syndrome youngsters have hassle adapting to exchange. Even a easy alternate in your each day recurring can purpose troubles. Although it's miles feasible to move correctly, you ought to devise nicely. This will ensure that the transition is smooth for actually each person. Your son, eleven years vintage, is aware and might recognize that there can be changes. This will no longer have an effect on how your son handles the alternate. These are some pointers to help you assume thru while you plan your subsequent bypass.

Tools to utilize

Pictures, visible aids-PECs gambling playing playing cards, pictures, visual schedules and aids will assist your son see what is taking region.

Social reminiscences-These recollections placed sports into written shape and are generally followed through pics.

Visitation-Plan visits to the new house, school, and network. Visits will help him turn out to be adjusted to these new places over time.

Sensory-New places have sincerely considered one of a kind moderate, uncommon smells, and new sounds. Blend the antique with the ultra-modern for the exceptional end result.

Your new home and college

Visual/Social Stories

Photograph your new college and domestic as regularly as viable. You can use the photographs to create an album approximately your new domestic. To create a social tale about your go with the flow, add clean captions. Give your son sufficient time to look through this album. Make some distinctive album, with pics of the university, the playground and the people. Include captions and names.

Visitation

Before the float, plan to go to your new residence Take a walk throughout the vicinity and experience the park Tell the owner/occupant about your scenario and ask if they will will assist you to go to the house in advance than the pass. Your son can take a look at the house and surrounding location to the photograph album. You can also speak the trends with him. Meet the workforce and visit the university. Take a excursion of the school and playground.

Sensory

Observe the sensory factors of the modern-day domestic and the encompassing community while you're there. It is essential to understand the sensory needs of your son. Does the residence smell unusual or wonderful? Before you skip in, make certain to hold the vintage household cleaners and air freshener in your new home. Make fantastic you take a look at the lighting fixtures. Is the sun shining in your son's mattress room on the same second in his new room? This need to help you decide the room your son may be the use of.

Keep subjects clean. Every infant is unique, so try and discover techniques to make your son satisfied. Your son's existence may be for all time modified by way of the steerage you're making.

Teenagers and Transition

five. How has Asperger's teens who went from junior immoderate to highschool completed? What come to be the finest mission?

Asperger's syndrome ought to have satisfied, a success immoderate college memories. A teen with Asperger's Syndrome can graduate excessive faculty and preserve directly to college in the event that they've the right plan.

Teens with Asperger's can face some unique challenges. Asperger's sufferers will every have their very own strengths and weaknesses. There are commonplace concerns for everybody on the Autism spectrum. These are some of the most common demanding situations confronted with the useful resource of teens with Asperger's Syndrome.

Communication problems-Communication might be the largest mission of Asperger's. The loss of ability to apprehend different people's body language and gestures, to make eye touch, and to approach language reasons hundreds frustration. This makes them come upon as aloof, or uncaring. On the indoors, they certainly need to be preferred and understood.

Change-Transitions are very hard for this organization. They are more cushty with a familiar regular, a fine order to matters, or a hard and speedy agenda. In high college, lifestyles is exchange. Everything movements at a faster pace and you're anticipated to go together with the glide. Kids unfold their wings at this age, getting jobs, developing specific pastimes, and forming precise

Peer relationships. Teens with Asperger's must be cautious within the ones regions.

Social reminiscences/Peer friendships-Making buddies and interacting with friends in social conditions may be painful critiques. High school is a very

social time and location. If you are not a player, you are in truth left at the back of. Teens with Asperger's use social skills training, counseling, and peer mentors to assist in social growth and development.

Obsessive pastimes-Sometimes those unique pursuits have a tendency to overrule all attempts at communication. People with Asperger's once in a while find it difficult to permit pass of these pastimes for the sake of shared verbal exchange. The truth is, they're inquisitive about the data and statistics of their obsession and that they do now not understand why others are not in addition enthralled.

Bullying-This is the most critical undertaking f or youngsters with Asperger's of every age. Bullying is privy to no barriers. Age does now not depend, social reputation is unimportant. Bullies pick out out their sufferers based totally totally totally on vulnerability. Kids with Asperger's are focused because of their awkwardness, obedience, and sensitivity. Parents ought to be active advocates to prevent bullying.

Teens with Asperger's Syndrome face many o ther demanding situations than the ones indexed right here. Teens with Asperger's can overcome those demanding situations and go directly to pursue exciting careers.

Chapter 2: New School Meltdowns

6. How can we address meltdowns inside the morning even as we start a contemporary Kindergarten and school?

Kindergarten is an indication of developing up. Your baby is now not a little one. It's a time of alternate! What is the greatest impediment for a younger Asperger's Syndrome toddler? Change.

Children with Asperger's are frequently frustrated thru the steady trade. Your toddler prospers at the equal time as there may be a set time table. He craves order and routine. If you allowed it, he would consume the right identical meals, located at the identical garments, play with the identical toys every day. This can motive tension and strain in the toddler, in addition to immoderate meltdowns. You can prepare your toddler for the adjustments in faculty.

Social stories

Carol Gray within the beginning created social stories. These memories describe an event or state of affairs in a easy, however clean manner it is smooth to comprehend. You can locate these tales in Mrs. Gray's books or create your personal. You can use pictures to create a social story to familiarize your infant's new university, instructor and study room.

Early instruction

Use your new social tale/image album to get started out making equipped your toddler for college. Arrange to take your toddler on a university tour and meet the teacher. It is a awesome concept to provide your toddler severa possibilities to excursion the faculty before college begins.

Visual time desk

Make a visible schedule of the day for your toddler. A seen time table includes pix, often PECs playing playing cards that depict the day's sports sports. Home schedules can embody wake-up time, dressing up, going to school, snack after school, play hobby, chore hobby and dinner. A college time desk can also encompass circle time and phonics, math snack, laptop time occupational remedy, lunch, naptime health club, circle time, easy up, and phonics.

Time

Sometimes, we surely want to preserve going and live affected person. After a time of adjustment, anxiety will begin to subside and faculty turns into ordinary. Your child can lighten up and enjoy the adventure with help from each university and home.

It is a ordinary a part of lifestyles, and also you need to embrace them. Your little one will quickly be a kindergarten seasoned, and your lifestyles will go lower back to everyday even as it is time for the subsequent step. These tools may be used to help your infant with Asperger's weather any transitions.

Making Friends in a New School

7. My granddaughter will begin university in September. Her most effective pal from nursery is transferring directly to some unique university. Without her great friend, she can be devastated. Are there any recommendations for a manner to deal with this?

A number one transition in a toddler's life can be starting college. Asperger's kids are sensitive to adjustments. Any disruption to a normal or schedule can reason a baby to revel in worrying. Your granddaughter had a a success and interesting three hundred and sixty five days at nursery. After she have become cushty with the contemporary regular and made friends, it become time to begin a current-day college one year. Children with Asperger's face the finest hassle in school: regular exchange.

These every 12 months modifications may be difficult, but they'll be triumph over. Although it'll probable be tough, your granddaughter will quickly adapt to her new college and find out a modern day pal. These are a few hints to assist your family cope with this example.

Advance Preparation

For a smooth transition, education is high. Asperger's children are visible. They like to investigate the information and information approximately any project don't forget or state of affairs. They are often referred to as "little professors". Tell your granddaughter all approximately the college year.

A social story about her university with images and real snap shots will provide her with a few factor to assess. She want to agenda a tour of the faculty and a meeting her new trainer. Photographs may be useful for her to refer again to often. Make a visible calendar to your granddaughter that lists all of the sports she may be taking part in among now and her first day at school. Discuss the modifications and the calendar often.

Therapy

In times of transition, treatment can show to be exceptionally useful. It can also marvel you to peer how your granddaughter adjusts to new university and new friends without feeling overwhelmed. Asperger's Syndrome youngsters are touchy and may be effects distracted thru new friends.

Children with Asperger's can seem properly-adjusted in such situations, no matter the truth that they will be truly struggling emotionally and devastation. Your granddaughter and her own family can benefit from man or woman, organization, or circle of relatives remedy with an Autism Spectrum Disorder counselor.

Your granddaughter's own family is aware of her more than genuinely absolutely everyone. You are familiar with the varieties of troubles that cause her issues. These issues may be addressed early in remedy and planning to make certain a clean transition.

What takes area if my toddler hates university?

eight. What can I do to begin my son's schoolyear on a fantastic be conscious after remaining one year complete of panic assaults, worry and rage? He hated college a lot that he refused to head. He was in a characteristic to finish his faculty yr at home. This is a exercising that I can not keep because of my art work time desk.

Your son appears like he has struggled at college. This is a problem that Asperger's Syndrome have to make more common. Asperger's children are smart however not one in every of a kind sufficient to be determined through their friends. They also are aware of their variations and want to sense regular. They do no longer understand that everyday is a relative idea as kids!

Although domestic education can be a top notch alternative for Asperger's Syndrome youngsters, it requires parental dedication and a whole lot of planning and time. Let's talk about methods to make your son's faculty enjoy higher.

Parent/teacher planning assembly

Meet with all university employees worried to your son's training. This organization should take transport of particular statistics approximately your son's evaluation, in addition to any emotional and scientific issues. Talk approximately viable issues that might prevent the college revel in for Asperger's Syndrome children. These embody bullying, boredom and the intensity of sophistication, assignments and the surroundings. To address those and distinct issues, create an Individual Education Plan (or IEP) collectively.

Parent/health practitioner making plans meeting

Now is the right time to tell your son's health practitioner approximately his struggles. These emotional troubles can cause bodily signs or maybe illness. It is critical to have a whole fitness checkup. If critical, communicate any health problems and capsules.

Parent/therapist planning assembly

An amazing counselor or therapist who is educated in Autism Spectrum problems can show to be very useful. Individual remedy can be beneficial to your son, similarly to circle of relatives or company lessons. Talk for your son about the ones options and any medicine that would assist him deal with his emotions. Although treatment is not right for everybody, it is able to be useful to your son to find out one of a kind alternatives.

Family planning assembly

As a family, sit down down and talk the residence regulations. It isn't an choice to skip to school. To ensure each person is aware about the effects of breaking residence tips, create a listing. You can help him make to-do lists, schedules and calendars. These visible aids will preserve his tension beneath manage. Your son need to recognize that you may approach his problems together.

There are many issues that your son need to cope with. He must be willing to art work hard to enhance his conduct. Your son can also want to have a first rate enjoy at university if he has a strong family assist and a clinical plan.

Education Strategies... How to Improve Time Management

nine. My 18-yr vintage son has Asperger's. His immoderate college schooling is on line via a charter university. He excels in university. He does now not realize the manner to govern his time and is constantly cramming for assignments. How can I help him manage his time in order that he can whole his assignments with out stress?

Procrastination is the worst thing that would do in your strain stages. Some humans are clearly procrastinators. Others, collectively together with your son, warfare to understand the concept of time. This is a not unusual characteristic of Asperger's Syndrome.

Teens with Asperger's can take online education. Your son's wondering techniques can be drastically improved if he is free of the distractions of school. There are many positives to don't forget: the lessening of sensory assault, one-on-one guidance, no bullies, and the bargain in sensory assault!

To prevent isolation, you may moreover recollect turning into a member of a social abilities organization or other social sports activities. He will gain from social abilties education in a comfortable surroundings thru becoming a member of golf equipment and community agencies that cater to his hobbies.

Many Asperger's children have a problem with organisation. Poor enterprise organisation can result in intense problems for Asperger's kids. Asperger's children are more likely to be troubled by using anxiety, depression, and strain. Young adults want to have organizational competencies. Students are anticipated to publish perfect art work on time via college and excessive college instructors. Positive adjustments can be made if you find out solutions now. These are a few strategies you could assist your son higher control his time.

Designing an ordered workspace is a fantastic place to start. A specific location for the whole thing, comfortable seating, quiet surroundings, and a calming decor will help lower distractions.

Creating a ordinary is important to your son. As someone with Asperger's is someone who craves order and ordinary. He may be capable of test a every day normal. To create a normal, he can also need a few guidance. You can paintings with him to make certain a easy float in his day.

Visual schedules are a crucial part of your son's regular. Use l ists and reminders to keep him shifting along. Encourage him to keep a each day, weekly, and month-to-month calendar. To do lists, written schedules, and project lists will supply him the form he wants to start organizing his life.

Visual timers may be very useful system at the same time as organizational skills are being taught. These timers have a coloured line that gets smaller because the time passes, giving the patron a actual visual photograph of strolling out of time. Each each day project or, to your son's case, every college issue, can be timed with the visual timer.

We are so glad with you for locating the solution for your son's university troubles. Teens with Asperger's Syndrome can discover immoderate faculty overwhelming. Your steering and organization will make sure that your son finishes high faculty with self perception and may move right now to maturity.

How can I inspire my infant to do university artwork?

10. My son, who has Asperger's, moreover has Tourette's. We in reality confirmed that he has focal seizures. He is not caused to move to school. He is a horrible scholar and

struggles to install writing. He sold a Neo2 word approach and wrote his first tale through himself. However, the novelty fast wore off and he failed to use it as an awful lot as we had was hoping for for his schoolwork. Are there any guidelines to encourage him to pay more attention and art work tougher?

The Neo2 is a first-rate tool to your son. It is important to no longer abandon the undertaking. He can also moreover quickly apprehend the advantages of the Neo2 for schoolwork if he has the right guide.

Your son has multiple scientific situations and Asperger's Syndrome. This is an sizeable burden for a child. His difficulty outcomes and extraordinary clinical situations need to make it difficult for him to popularity on schoolwork. It's clean to count on that college ought to overwhelm a little one alongside collectively with his scientific conditions.

Chapter 3: Special Education

Ask for a assembly with the training crew of your son. For assessment, cutting-edge clinical records together with medicines and diagnoses need to be furnished. For instructional reviews, request a present day day one. Remind your trainer approximately the significance of imparting emotional useful resource as well as academic help.

You want to revise your son's IEP to consist of recent scientific conditions and evaluations, in addition to allow the usage of special augmentative devices much like the Neo2. You can now request any versions that your son might also require. Common versions in training plans embody greater checking out time and decreased writing workload.

Special pastimes

Encourage your son's hobby in his interests and pursuits. Asperger's children will be inclined to be obsessive approximately positive pastimes. You can use his pastimes to encourage him to finish his schoolwork. He might be happier and greater engaged if he has first-rate social studies alongside along with his pals and circle of relatives.

Special equipment

Your son could be able to control his day with calm and competence if you provide him the proper machine. Asperger's disease is commonplace and might reason tension, pressure, and lack of motivation. You can assist him make lists and create schedules to perform his daily duties. He can revel in greater on pinnacle of factors thru developing visible schedules for his college assignments, every day chores, in addition to his at-home recurring.

Your son can attain college if he has the right educational, clinical, and emotional useful resource. A plan that addresses maximum of these regions will beautify your son's motivation and eliminate some of the stress you have got all been sporting.

Need assist with Test

11. My eighth grade son goals help with his exams. He forgets to write down his name, skips questions, and would not proofread his paintings. He often gets factors for incorrect answers to brief solution questions. Can you please advocate?

Asperger's youngsters are greater at risk of pressure and tension than exclusive kids and can warfare with changes. Your son can also moreover moreover feel emotional ache if there are any changes to his every day habitual.

Asperger's Syndrome kids can sense beaten even as taking assessments. It isn't always common for children with Asperger's Syndrome to take assessments every day. Testing is regularly timed, that can upload stress and anxiety. You can help your son at home and you need to do the same for him at school. This will make his day greater effective.

At Home

Your son can also want help organizing his thoughts. A written plan is vital on your son for you to use in disturbing conditions. He desires to make a listing of things that want to be achieved on test day. The listing may be quite precise. It can also moreover start with getting a first-rate night time's sleep the night time in advance than. Here's an instance of a check software:

1.Good night time time's sleep

2. Eat an notable breakfast

three. Arrive on time-no dashing!

four. Put your call on paper. Do this as speedy to procure your paper!

five. Pay attention to the commands of your teacher

6. Each query have to be checked for the solution. Did you pass over any questions?

7. Each solution is a whole sentence? 8. Always proofread if you have the time.These lists need for use at the same time as

organization is a problem. Your son can be prepared with each day lists, calendar pages, or written schedules. His organizing gadget will assist him recognize what to expect every day. This will lessen strain and tension.

At School

Any troubles which might be causing troubles in college have to be addressed by way of way of your son's person education plan (IEP). An IEP will often encompass take a look at troubles. You must make precise arrangements in your son, together with extra time or custom designed assistance in some unspecified time in the future of attempting out. An aide can be available to useful useful resource him in some unspecified time in the future of trying out.

Talk in your son's college organization approximately those troubles similarly to each exclusive issues he may be having at college. You can allow them to recognize that even as you work on company at home, you experience that he however desires extra guide at university. Be open to the guidelines of the school frame of personnel and listen on your personal thoughts. A supportive, encouraging and willing to art work together to advantage the solutions your son goals is top to his success at college.

How can I inspire my son to transport outside?

12. My son prefers to examine and stand in area of participate in outdoor prepared video games. His slow response time and clumsiness also can provide an reason for some of his hesitation. How can I encourage him to participate and revel in those activities with me?

Asperger's Syndrome kids discover organized sports and video video games difficult. They seem to deal with every issue of Asperger's Syndrome, along side social talents, sensory troubles, coordination troubles, and physical awkwardness. Your son may be reluctant to participate. He desires to have the possibility to play in outdoor and institution sports activities sports to overcome the Asperger's symptoms. Below is a listing of viable alternatives and a few pointers for encouraging Asperger's kids to strive physical activities.

Family sports activities sports and video games are a wonderful location to start. Family individuals are greater tolerant and forgiving of each one of a kind's faults. Playing video games with the own family will improve your son's self guarantee. This can also even permit him time to look at suggestions and movements on the way to make him a fulfillment at the video video video games he chooses to try.

Recreational sports activities sports sports activities and video video games are generally provided to your network with the beneficial resource of city parks and close by church homes. These leagues or businesses recognition on education kids to play video video games and sports successfully, nicely teamwork, and team spirit. There is mostly a desire to win, however the ones leagues emphasize appropriate sportsmanship over winning. Here you may discover the brought manual your son desires to interrupt into institution video games or sports. Competitive sports and video video games can be attempted as quickly as your son is assured in his functionality to play the sport and snug at the social degree. Some kids also can in no way play competitively and this is ok.

But do no longer restriction your son's participation in amusement leagues. Let your son make the final choice. Many Asperger's kids can compete on the high degree of competition without hassle.

Your son can be overly concerned together together with his coordination or clumsiness. An individual lacking in social abilties can result in anxiety and embarrassment on the smallest of missteps. You might not apprehend how deep the ones feelings can run. Therapy can be completed beforehand of time.

Psychological therapy-individual remedy will help you son address regular life, awful emotions, stress, and tension.

Physical treatment-An evaluation with a certified bodily therapist will display physical troubles that can be corrected thru remedy.

Social talents remedy-This remedy is generally held in corporations to facilitate

social situations with steerage. Children with Asperger's learn how to

relate to others socially throughout those commands.

Remember that now not every person are inquisitive about outside and sports sports sports activities activities. You son might likely have other hobbies which might be more pleasing. No depend what he does alongside together with his unfastened time, it's far critical that he feels supported and loved with the aid of way of his circle of relatives.

How can I get my son's trainer to pay interest!

thirteen. How can I get instructors and public colleges to be aware of my son and to surely take delivery of his instructional and emotional needs?

Asperger's Syndrome may be a complex circumstance. Each Asperger's little one has his or her private particular scenario. Asperger's children are realistic and function a number of capacity for studying. A toddler could probably have hassle reading however be very talented in math. Teachers may additionally furthermore query the validity of clinical diagnoses because of the fact they're now not capable of understand the unbalanced abilties and immoderate intelligence that lead to school troubles.

Except for the ones who've studied special schooling, public faculty teachers are anticipated to train regular kids. It is unreasonable to expect that every one instructors may be able to apprehend all the developmental and neurological problems that may upward thrust up inside the classroom.

Public and public education about Asperger's Syndrome is in top notch name for. It is crucial that your son's college be knowledgeable approximately Asperger's and the way it impacts him at university.

These are a few useful recommendations for this education.

Local Autism help organisation observed out records-Provide facts approximately Asperger's Syndrome and the signs and symptoms it reasons. Use statistics that is direct and to-the-problem. Highlight the areas in which your son has weak point. Also, highlight his strengths.

Medical statistics: Neurological testing, proof of bodily health, psychological sorting out, and any medicinal capsules used (and why) are critical facts that the university must keep in mind. Have your son's doctors write letters explaining any physical or emotional issues for which he's handled and the way they will have an effect on him at university.

Occupational treatment opinions-These documents will encompass your son's sensory eating regimen, which is what he desires to fight sensory troubles on a each day basis.

Physical treatment critiques-These documents will encompass data on physical issues you son desires to paintings on and the manner the deficits should have an impact on his faculty day.

Speech/Language treatment evaluations-Speech remedy is a lot greater than articulation. These files will consist of a plan that tackles language processing issues and social skills goals, further to many distinct possible troubles.

Educational evaluations may be done thru your son's training employer. These reviews also can or may not healthy yours. You need to be your son's endorse and look at all criminal steps to make sure his success in college. Your son's individual education plan (IEP) want to cope with all issues that cause troubles at college. You can determine what is remarkable on your toddler and the manner a long manner you may go to ensure that the school troubles are addressed.

Why does my daughter play with greater younger children?

14. My daughter will input 1/3 grade in the fall. She prefers to play at recess with greater youthful boys and ignores women in her elegance. What can I do to get my daughter to play collectively along with her grade-degree girl buddies at recess?

Asperger's Syndrome kids frequently gravitate to extra younger children. Your daughter also can favor to play with extra younger boys than her friends for hundreds of reasons. Let's test some of the motives.

Peer pain

Social play is a fave interest for girls. Classic female video video video games embody mommy and toddler dolls and instructor, scholar, medical doctor, and affected man or woman. These video games include quite a few pretending and plenty of social verbal exchange.

Asperger's Syndrome youngsters may additionally moreover moreover have hassle with faux play and social interaction. To break out social pressures, your daughter might be looking to keep away from her woman pals.

Bullying

Experts document that nearly all Asperger's children are bullied at one time or a few one of a kind inside the path in their college years. This is a sad reality. Bullies can come at any age, be boys or girls, and cause great soreness. Maybe your daughter has been bullied thru her woman friends.

Social immaturity Asperger's youngsters are often a bit too younger for his or her age in social sports. This is regularly the number one signal that there may be a hassle. A infant who isn't always mature will clearly gravitate to youngsters with similar maturity. Boys will be inclined to play greater socially, which makes it lots less difficult in your toddler to control that detail of play.

Parallel play

Your daughter may be playing with the more youthful boys, as opposed to with them. This can be very not unusual in Asperger's. This lets in your daughter to play with more youthful boys without any social involvement.

Let's now look at the viable reasons of your daughter's conduct.

Parent/instructor involvement

To talk your issues, time table a assembly with the trainer of your daughter. To rule out bullying, you have got to test out the issue. Talk approximately the way you trust you studied your daughter should be socially stretched, inner her consolation degree, in order to conquer her troubles together with her peers. Ask for particular services and remedy plans to help.

Social talents education

Your daughter can benefit from social abilties treatment to enhance her potential to talk and relate with others, along with her friends. Although those training aren't furnished in every college, most community manual companies offer social competencies training. You may be capable of find out distinctive commands on your close by vicinity through your daughter's psychologist or health practitioner.

Chapter 4: Peer Mentoring

Peer-mentoring is gaining recognition. It pairs an Asperger's infant with a neurotypical peer to mentor in the course of college hours. The peer-mentoring software program application is based totally totally on the children's grades, behavior, and person.

These issues can be addressed and your daughter will revel in extra comfortable. Your daughter's happiness can be a key component of her development. As you push her to the boundaries, hold her comfortable degree in thoughts.

My five 12 months vintage Daughter is Scared of School artwork

15. My 5-12 months-vintage daughter does no longer need to do her homework. Although she claims she is afraid or not able to do the art work, all of us realise that she will be able to. How can teachers and I get her running on her assignments while she's required?

Your daughter is five years vintage and but a newcomer to high school. Asperger's Syndrome ought to make it tough for youngsters to modify to being new. Asperger's Syndrome youngsters aren't capable of cope with trade well. They pick habitual and order. Your daughter can be afraid if she says so. This is because of the truth she is telling you that it is new for her and is frightening. These are some tips that might assist you to ease your daughter's transition.

Routine and order are very crucial to children with Asperger's Syndrome. Feelings of worry and lack of ability are right away associated with your daughter's enjoy of feeling out of manipulate. Creating a every day routine will deliver your daughter a feel of manage and luxury. Once she is privy to what to anticipate in all situations, she can be capable of perform to meet her capabilities.

Schedules and lists are very useful seen aids for youngsters with Asperger's. A photo agenda will allow your daughter to look precisely what is predicted in some unspecified time in the future of the college day. Fewer surprises suggest higher edition. An example would be the ones classes: circle time, reading, snack, fitness center, lunch, naptime, math, pc, and clean up. Each beauty may want to have a corresponding picture. Some schedules have a laminated photograph of the kid that can be moved to each elegance due to the fact the day progresses.

Intelligence and talents may also come into play on a every day foundation.

You, as her mom, realise exactly what your daughter can do.

can see. When feasible, encourage your daughter to pursue her precise pastimes. Your daughter's preference to research greater approximately her pastimes will help her to be higher informed. Keep reminding her that she is wise and succesful.

Therapies are frequently preferred for youngsters with Asperger's. The without a doubt one among a kind specialists at college can deal with your daughter's speech/language deficits, her sensory and motor capabilities desires, any coordination issues that could interfere with college success, and her social abilities requirements.

IEP dreams and specific interest may be very beneficial for a kid with Asperger's. If you have not already, request an man or woman education plan in your daughter. Her scientific and academic evaluations will help the organization shape a plan on the way to tools her for success. Other than the treatments referred to above, you could want to indicate decreased homework, extra time for seat artwork and assessments, particular seating area inside the look at room, and if important, a one-on-one aide to provide assist all through the day.

Your daughter will blossom once the transition is entire. Your daughter may be in a role to show her intelligence and advantage self notion. It may not be smooth. Keep these thoughts in mind so your daughter can adapt to new conditions.

How can I help my Child's Organization Skills

16. How are we able to assist Asperger's children apprehend the importance of organization?

Organization is crucial in every issue of life. Asperger's Syndrome children have hassle studying this skills. Unorganized intelligence ought to make even the brightest infant appear silly. You can train Asperger's Syndrome on your toddler purposeful organizational competencies.

It is feasible that your toddler will not apprehend the importance of corporation, specifically if it is an inherent a part of his personality. Sometimes people clearly have an unintended tendency to be messy. There is a possibility that you can have a double disease. Here are a few thoughts to help you teach organizational competencies.

Slow and constant, brief steps

It is top notch to take it step by step. Select the problem place that requires improvement. You can destroy it down into schooling or quick corrections. If your infant is liable to forgetting homework, you could help him amplify a tool a good way to not fail. To save you any out of vicinity or forgotten work, a folder may be used to document his assignments. It also can be used to move his work among college and home. Give yourself loads of time for strong improvement in advance than you pass on to the following place. Slow and constant wins. Your toddler will test speedy and take small steps to keep the race from becoming overwhelming.

Visual and tested, proof and reward

Asperger's Syndrome youngsters are quite visual. Visual capabilities need to be used on every occasion possible. Written lists, calendars, schedules, and terrific system can all be used to help your infant stay organized. Teachers regularly use photograph schedules to assist kids hold music in their chores and other every day duties. Encourage your little one to apply visible aids just like the ones. Praise them for following a agenda or list. Organization is critical for achievement. This will result in better grades and lots much less stress. Applauding others will help to validate their efforts and encourage future ones.

Last but now not least, ask your baby's instructors for help in explaining the importance of agency capabilities and education them a way to use them. Asperger's kids need consistency in their getting to know. Repeating college and home training will help you emphasize the importance of organization. In future Asperger's sports sports, the parent/trainer institution can be a precious useful beneficial useful resource.

Reading, Writing and Spelling Methods

17. How can I train my thirteen-year vintage son to spell, take a look at and write? In the beyond, unique training have no longer helped.

Asperger's Syndrome youngsters frequently find out university a supply for frustration. Asperger's Syndrome can purpose troubles with conversation, comprehension, and auditory analyzing. Often, horrible high-quality motor abilities avoid handwriting development. These troubles can cause studying problems and frustration. This frustration can reason stress and tension that could result in horrible instructional outcomes.

Asperger's children have their private strengths and weaknesses. It is important that you amplify an academic plan that fits your son's goals. These are a few thoughts and ideas approximately schooling and schooling spelling, writing, and studying.

Special Education

Even in case your enjoy with particular training become awful, there are legal hints that shield your son's right for a loose and appropriate public schooling. You have the proper not to surrender on precise training. You can maintain attempting one-of-a-kind instructors and remedy plans until you find out the first rate one. You can similarly your training through way of searching IDEA and FAPE, Wright's Law and IEP to your specific usa.

Home Schooling

Many mother and father with Asperger's youngsters homeschool their youngsters. This calls for loads of time, effort, cash, and strength of mind. There are many websites devoted to homeschooling special dreams children. There are help groups for households who want to start their adventure. Ask your nearby librarian approximately home schooling, and what requirements your kingdom has. National group, the Home School Legal Defense

Association (HSLDA), informs people approximately their rights in regards to domestic schooling particular education and homeschooling in massive.

Teaching Approaches and Ideas Although phonics is the maximum commonplace way to train analyzing, it does no longer art work for all. Children with unique wishes might also additionally find out the whole word approach to be fairly effective. Asperger's children are visible beginners. Instead of starting with sounds and letters, start with phrases. For extra visible enchantment and impact, encompass photographs. Make it fun and keep the instructions quick.

The fine manner to educate Asperger's children to examine, spell and write is to pay interest on their unique pastimes. This will permit them in case you want to contain all subjects. If your son is interested in sports activities sports cars, you could have a take a look at books about them with him, following his lead. To help decorate writing capabilities, have him draw or hint motors.

Create playing cards with automobile pics and upload one word from the tale to each. These may be used as flashcards and you could studies the words via setting them inside the story order. To educate spelling, you can use the terms within the story. Draw a photo of your son that lets in him take into account the word. Ask him to pick out out someone from the story after which write a paragraph.

Every week, find out a extraordinary story to entertain and inspire your son. Begin with smooth testimonies, and then bypass straight away to more complex tales. This method may be used to educate your son about any problem. Have amusing!

How can I get my son to study the trainer's commands?

18. How can I get my son understand that he have to look at the teacher's instructions to complete the hassle earlier than him, in

desire to thrilling the children around him or taking over a few different state of affairs just because of the reality he believes he can do it at domestic?

Asperger's Syndrome can motive children to exhibit behavioral problems in faculty environments. Asperger's Syndrome can now and again avoid a child's capability to act in a responsible way. This makes the college day difficult for children with Asperger's. Every toddler with Asperger's can also additionally have his or her private precise state of affairs. These consist of obsessive preoccupations, sensory issues, horrible social abilties, the want to be habitual, sameness and order, terrible motor competencies (outstanding and gross), auditory processing problems, comprehension struggles, and the tendency toward anxiety and melancholy.

These complicated traits mean that there may be nobody manner to cope with conduct issues. To be capable of comply along with his personal education plan, every pupil should have a custom designed plan for conduct. Your son's IEP or man or woman schooling plan want to encompass behavioral issues. Your son will conflict to have a examine if he may no longer have behavioral guide. These are only some recommendations.

IEP changesIt may be time to time table a assembly together together with your son's education crew. Request a state-of-the-art behavioral assessment to find out the areas of discord in the classroom. The behavioral assessment also can display your son's sensory troubles are immoderate, for example. With this data, the team can extend a plan to keep away from sensory overload.

Parent/trainer relationshipBe a strong excellent pal in the quest on your son's schooling. His trainer wishes his success as a good buy as you do. Work together to form a strong place plan, in which desired. Clowning should no longer be tolerated. Talk regularly to maintain all of us knowledgeable on changes at home that would cause problems at university.

Rules, schedules, physical video games-These are all crucial for appropriate conduct. Your son desires the form those gear provide. Keep written lists of policies, chores, schedules, and expectations for domestic and for college visible every time possible. Routines are critical. Even a tiny trade in routine can cause behavioral problems. It is difficult for your son to truly accept and modify to those modifications.

Preventing issues conduct is the important element to higher observe room behavior. Your son will behave properly with the useful resource he gets at university and home. You can inspire your son to be higher, no longer tremendous by way of manner of teaching new behaviors and punishing him, however also via retaining off worrying conditions.

My Son roams for the duration of the School

19. My son is now in Grade 1. He observed out to sit down down and entire his responsibilities.

Sometimes he wanders at some stage in the college, from time to time leaving the school room. This takes vicinity approximately once consistent with week. What can I do to inspire him?

Your son may be capable of alter to highschool existence after a year. This is why many more youthful Asperger's Syndrome youngsters do nicely at school. Your son will experience more cushty in elegance if the time table is everyday at this grade diploma. There are sports activities whilst the agenda might trade a piece or the noise degree is probably better than commonplace. These are matters we won't phrase but need to reason sufficient ache in your son to need to escape.

It can be very troubling that your son leaves the lecture room so often without being supervised. The college need to cope with this trouble. It is a exquisite concept to inspire your son to obey college tips and stay in his look at room, however the hassle is some distance extra intense than you located. These are a few approaches to cope with this complex situation.

Staff schooling Asperger's Syndrome can be a complex scenario. To speak the situation in your son's university, meet with the precept. Give statistics approximately Asperger's to give an reason for why your son feels the need to flee. Talk approximately the risks. Staff should be informed about Asperger's Syndrome, and the manner it impacts your infant.

IEP

To revise your son's IEP, or person education plan, invite his academic group to meet with you. Your son's teacher may be conscious that he is leaving college. There are extra important problems if she is not aware. This scenario can be controlled with the aid of manner of using the trainer, however college safeguards must be in region to save you it from taking place. As the instructor isn't always able to manage the situation, you have to request an aide. Request a opportunity teacher if crucial.

It is a good idea to invite for up to date critiques and assessments. An assessment of behavior can also help to pinpoint the reasons why your son is trying to flee so you can create a preventative software software.

Visual Aids Visual schedules are beneficial at university and domestic. To create a day by day time desk board, use images of college subjects and sports activities. So your son is aware of even as his next ruin is coming, encompass snack, lunch, recess and lunch. To make sure continuity, create a time table just like your own home sports.

Asperger's kids have robust instincts to comply with the tips. To illustrate each rule, create a visible rule ebook the usage of easy images and written policies. This list may be used to remind your son not to leave the observe room.

While you can assist your son understand why he must live in his have a study room, the teacher is responsible for this. Press your son's college to recovery the trouble in his examine room.

Too hundreds spare time at School

20. My son has an excessive amount of free time. He does no longer see this as his time for studying. How can I get him a one-of-a-type mind-set and permit him to apply his time to gain his marks?

Asperger's syndrome youngsters need to balance their obligations. They need to face up to the urge to dive headfirst into their obsessions or to isolate themselves from others. Because business enterprise and time control are not their robust suits, they may lose tune of the time. Your son's passions will frequently overshadow the significance of schoolwork, specifically while he has more time to indulge.

It can be hard to assist your son recognize that he goals extra check time. These are my mind on priorities, corporation and Asperger's Syndrome.

Special pastimes vs. School paintings

One or of his maximum excessive pastimes are all-eating. These hobbies are his number one reputation and he is probably content material cloth to spend all of his waking hours pursuing them. This is a everyday function of Asperger's Syndrome. This isn't to reason inflammation. Finding a connection with your special hobby is the vital detail to schoolwork. Let's assume your son is captivated with biology and wants to come to be a biologist. It is crucial to have a stable education. This ought to inspire him to art work difficult to collect the grades he requires to recognize his dreams.

Spare time and isolation

Asperger's Syndrome patients ought to now not waste time. Boredom and despair can end result from a lack of hours. Your son may additionally furthermore end up depressed and remoted, that could reason anxiety or even despair, that could bring about extreme troubles. You have to right now take movement if your son starts offevolved to avoid college or is preoccupied through a selected interest. Encourage him to get involved with others and to are looking for counseling to assist alongside alongside with his melancholy and isolation.

Organization

Encourage your son to be prepared is the best detail you can do. This is each other important Asperger's characteristic-disorganization. Your son can control his time with seen aids together with 'first and remaining' charts, study plans, and every day schedules that include have a examine and precise pastimes.

To ensure a wholesome body and thoughts, encourage your son to stability art work, play, social sports, on my own time, and family time. Your son will fast research the significance of organisation and be capable of find the time to do the subjects which might be important to him in addition to the subjects that interest him.

My Son won't edit his School Work

21. How can I get my little one another time to highschool and ensure he's accurate? His instructor asks him to test the paintings and accurate any errors. He refuses to do this. He informs her that he is completed.

When it entails schoolwork, children can be particularly impatient. It can be worrying to finish an project pleasant to want to go back to check the complete task. This method should learn how to all youngsters, no longer honestly humans with Asperger's Syndrome. This and exclusive organizational talents are areas that maximum Asperger's kids have trouble with.

Your baby's rigid questioning is every different problem. Asperger's children are regularly inflexible in their wondering and inflexible in all conditions. It may be tough to trade their mind. Rigidity is a way to cope with uncomfortable situations. This is a few difficulty which you need to accept and artwork to rectify.

Therapy is always endorsed. Individual treatment plans that deal with sensory issues, communication, emotion, social capabilities, verbal exchange and verbal exchange are all useful to youngsters with Asperger's. You also can artwork on excellent abilties at domestic. These are only a few pointers to help you get started out out.

Control that rigid thinking. As tough because it sounds, your infant wants to find out about flexibility. Tiny agenda adjustments, like a snack in advance than nap in desire to the normal nap and then snack, can inspire bendy questioning. There are instances when even tiny changes might be too much. These checks need to be practiced on specific days.

Social recollections to the rescue! Find or create social testimonies about youngsters Use the talents that you are strengthening. Tell a story approximately a baby who takes a take a look at and goes again to affirm his answers. Explain in element how the child may enjoy, and supply an purpose of that it is suitable to now not do a critical challenge.

Make it part of his recurring. Routines are important to youngsters with Asperger's. By along with proofreading to your child's routine at domestic and at school, you may be growing a present day addiction.

Put it on the time table. Add "check your art work" reminders for your infant' s written each day time desk, sincerely as you encompass meal instances and sleep times. Your baby will need to proofread his artwork to move on thru his daily time table.

Rules are intended to be observed. Better but, make it a rule to proofread, no exceptions. Your infant has a herbal desire to conform with the hints and do the proper thing because of Asperger's.

Remember to consist of your toddler's training department while you are coping with issues that could have an impact on university average overall performance. These techniques must be carried out via the university team of workers in collaboration with you. This will help your infant emerge as a successful scholar at faculty and in lifestyles.

Educating your little one's university... Principal Says my Child can not Learn

22. The number one of the college has been stopping me each step of the manner. These kids, she says, cannot look at. My son is capable of observe English and Spanish, and he can also write a hint. He does not communicate. I sincerely have a question: Are those youngsters capable to investigate and excel at college?

Asperger's and Autism Spectrum Disorder children can excel in college, college and ordinary life. Don't permit the principle convince you otherwise. Your son is entitled to take part in normal college as tons as his capability will permit. Autism Spectrum children are frequently capable of whole-time inclusion. This trouble is blanketed via IDEA, the Individuals with Disabilities Education Act. IDEA changed into created to make certain people with disabilities have get right of get right of entry to to to a unfastened, suitable public education (FAPE), in the most restrictive setting possible.

It is antique questioning to strain children with special goals into self-contained precise training training. To inspire your son's boom and improvement, you must cope with him as an equal alongside along with his pals. Autism education is a essential want in this faculty. It's time to act. These are just a few tips. Request a alternate for your son's placement in a letter to the fundamental.

Make positive to copy the school tool's unique education coordinator and some extraordinary man or woman of interest. Request a response in writing. Do now not be afraid to cite all over again any remarks to the most. Say some aspect like, "Just to make sure I understand, you said that my son should now not be located in a ordinary classroom because of the fact kids like him aren't able to studying. Is this what you supposed?" Keep notes of all feedback and conversations for future reference.

Request an IEP meeting to speak about revision of your son's IEP. Insist that the meeting be scheduled at a time on hand for the critical and the unique desires coordinator to wait. If viable, locate an Autism advocacy group that offers IEP assist. Make a request for inclusion, unique concessions like greater time and decreased workload, and a whole time aide, if essential.

This precept has made derogatory remarks that show her lack of knowledge concerning unique training and autism spectrum conditions. In addition, her feedback are unwarranted and fake. This is discriminatory and judgmental. A strongly worded letter to the superintendent and the board of schooling is advocated to record this incident and any others.

Don't take delivery of much less together with your son. You apprehend your son better than certainly every body. You are capable of discover his strengths and weaknesses in addition to his capability. Signing an IEP that isn't to your son's wonderful pursuits need to be averted. You ought to make an effort to test the desires and offerings. Don't be afraid to carry it lower lower back to the desk until you're happy that the plan is appropriate on your son's public training.

How can I introduce my little one's new teacher to him?

23. How can I introduce my child's new instructor to him? Last three hundred and sixty five days, we wrote an advent letter with

a image and stored a pocket ebook that contained his diagnosis and advised movements. It by no means were given examine, I count on. Perhaps it changed into an excessive amount of records for an already overburdened teacher. How can I permit my son's classmates and extraordinary pals within the take a look at room apprehend his "distinction", simply so they do not get mad at him or tease him?

Teachers are trouble to quite a few expectations. In some cases, the study room may additionally encompass as many as thirty college college students. Some college college students may additionally additionally moreover need unique care. This is a huge duty that consists of a modest financial praise. Teachers frequently spend their very personal cash to inventory their study room with the whole lot, from pencils and papers to band-aids to greater garb.

It is useful to have precise data about a student's instructional, scientific or emotional desires. However, it may be overwhelming for teachers who're making geared up to spend the following 9-to twelve months with a latest magnificence of university students. These are some tips for the manner to introduce your son to his new instructor and fellow classmates.

An introductory letter is a tremendous idea. The key is to preserve it short and easy. The instructor does not have time to look at a medical mag description of Autism. A onepage precis of your son's strengths and weaknesses associated with Asperger's Syndrome (and every other clinical conditions) can be informative and beneficial to the trainer. The instructor is more likely to observe and refer returned to a brief summary than a

specific pocket book.

Contact your son's college and ask to satisfy his instructor in advance than college starts offevolved offevolved. This will offer you with a threat to supply the introductory letter and to reply any questions the instructor may also have. Giving your son a sneak peek so you can preserve to put together him for the imminent modifications he will quickly enjoy is an introduced bonus.

Ask to cope with the beauty on your son's behalf early inside the college 3 hundred and sixty five days. Explain Asperger's Syndrome on your son's classmates in a top notch mild. Talk about how Asperger's impacts your son in particular. Explain that he might also additionally get definitely disappointed if recess is cancelled, that he might also moreover speak an excessive amount of at the wrong instances, and that he has hassle taking turns. Ask the youngsters to assist your son be the incredible he may be each day. You may be amazed at how well university progresses after this speak.

Request that the employees analyze approximately Autism and Asperger's Syndrome. The university's psychologist can help, further to the occupational and physical therapists. Most instructors take minimal particular education guides and will welcome an informative meeting so one can supply them statistics they are able to use in the have a look at room this yr and in years to come.

These steps will beautify the connection amongst discern and instructor, as well as facilitate a clean transition for your little one's go again to highschool. Teachers understand mother and father who are concerned and knowledgeable. Parents moreover apprehend informed and involved teachers.

Chapter 5: Changing School Mindset

24. My twelve-12 months-vintage infant is at college at least as soon as every week. How are you able to with politeness tell the college that this little one has a disability and no longer be disrespectful? It can be hard to alternate this thoughts-set.

Many educators omit out at the link among behavior troubles and disability. Children are unpredictable and can create new and sudden situations every day. Every student has a right to an off day. Why want to Asperger's Syndrome college college students be any exquisite? Every little one has moments of disobedience and disregard. Educators need to type via those conditions and determine a manner to preserve - to punish or to pardon.

It becomes less tough to apprehend why your infant can also additionally adopt a horrible outlook while you keep in mind the severa examples of terrible conduct that educators have visible. This does no longer help if it's miles your infant who has legitimate motives for his behavior.

Asperger's Syndrome kids face many demanding situations in school. Many of those barriers can bring about conduct troubles. Asperger's can reason behavior troubles by using manner of inflicting a lack of communique, social competencies, or cognitive competencies. Prevention is the important thing to higher conduct. These are some strategies you could help your son and a few guidelines to help you address his teachers.

Cognitive-behavioral remedy-This remedy can help your son learn how to cope better via using dealing with his emotions and rigid questioning, among one of a kind issues. Appropriate behaviors also are cited and practiced at a few degree within the ones periods.

Social skills remedy-This company remedy encourages social interplay in a managed setting with a therapist acting as a facilitator.

Improved social skills can assist your son avoid some horrible conditions within the observe room.

Speech/communication therapy-This treatment works on improving twoway verbal exchange and any articulation issues.

Social testimonies-These tales can be used to talk about suitable reactions and behaviors in plenty of conditions. You can locate social tales on line, in books, or you could create your private. Social testimonies in comedian form are in particular well-known on your son's age institution.

Parent/teacher relationships-It may be very vital which you come to be an worried team member. Request conferences in conjunction with your son's instructors and shape a recreation plan, collectively, so that you can address his conduct troubles.

School frame of employees trainingYour son's educators need to realize the facts about Asperger's Syndrome. Supply the university with educational substances that specify the symptoms and signs and symptoms and signs and signs of Asperger's, together with the recommended treatments.

IEP behavioral plan-Your son desires a behavioral plan blanketed in his individualized education plan (IEP). Request an IEP assembly for revisions.

Parents of children with Asperger's Syndrome should not need to move to highschool every week because of conduct issues. Teamwork can assist beautify the state of affairs. Talking approximately the state of affairs and then imposing a plan is a manner to benefit your university and your son.

School Refusing to Help

25. How are you able to convince teachers and principals to deliver your little one more educational assist in areas in which they're struggling?

Asperger's Syndrome can be a complex condition. Your toddler seems to be regular on many levels. He is sensible and speaks in a way which makes him seem mature and vivid. He makes first-rate impressions on adults and is more comfortable spherical them. When he's collectively along with his buddies, his issues are multifaceted.

Parents can't control the moves and thoughts of community educators. As a figure of a little one identified with Asperger's Syndrome, you've got the obligation and the right to recommend for the manual offerings your infant requires to gain university. These are a few guidelines to help you get began.

Parent/teacher meeting

It is a exceptional concept to invite your little one's trainer to fulfill you. Be organized to talk approximately your problems approximately your little one's educational ordinary normal overall performance. You can take a list of the issues you have got decided and write it down. As a take a look at, talk possible help in the take a look at room to peer if she advantages. You may be more likely to get preserve of her cooperation in case you assemble an great relationship.

Special desires coordinator meeting

Next, meet with the college's unique schooling coordinator. You can take the notes from the teacher assembly and invite the instructor. Discuss with your son his instructional weaknesses.

Written request for opinions Send a right request for critiques for your college essential or unique goals coordinator.

Physician's letter and referrals

Ask your toddler's doctor for help via asking for a request letter requesting critiques. Ask your son to offer data if he has been identified with Asperger's Syndrome. Referrals to a personal psychologist or neurologist might be made for critiques. Your evaluation effects aren't required through the college system. However, they'll help you to take into account your next steps if essential.

Local Disabilities Services and Advocacy corporations

For facts about autism offerings and advocates, touch your neighborhood Autism assist employer. They will assist you to apprehend your rights. You have the proper to big schooling. If you are recognized with Asperger's Syndrome, there are federal and state prison hints an great way to shield you. You have to make an effort to have a look at precise schooling regulation, specifically IDEA (the Individuals with Disabilities Education Act).

Your son can be extra a success at university if he has the right guide. Your son's faculty personnel can be more statistics if they're informed.

Other Education Issues... School Bullying

26. My son, who's now in secondary college, has had problems because he moved there very last twelve months. My son grow to be bullied lots that he refused to take the

university bus. He is now taking his husband to high school each morning, however we generally inform him that he's going to get the bus all another time for the second year. He will probable panic even as that thing comes and refuse to adventure the bus. However, if we permit him to pressure to highschool, it's going to make it even extra hard to get him once more on the bus. I need some advice on the manner to cope with the strain?

Children with Asperger's Syndrome are regularly assignment to bullying. This can reason tension and pressure. Bullying is so not unusual, a few professionals recall that the majority kids with Asperger's revel in it. Bullies love children with Asperger's due to the fact they discover them unique enough. Although most faculties have guidelines toward bullying, it could be difficult to put into impact them. Teachers and dad and mom may not recognize that a infant with Asperger's is being bullied due to their communication troubles.

You have found out that being aware about the scenario isn't always a guarantee for a powerful final effects. The bullying revel in your son has expert motives him immoderate stress and anxiety, that would negatively impact his fitness and properly-being. Negative research can cause strain in his lifestyles and cause him to war. These are some recommendations for a manner to control this case. School manage assembly

Ask for a meeting with the school personnel. All times of bullying want to be said to the university. You have to make a formal complaint in your school and ask them that will help you treatment the bullying problem on the bus to your son.

Therapy and medication

These occasions have had a terrible impact on your son. Individual remedy or remedy that reduces stress, tension, panic, and different symptoms and symptoms can be beneficial on your son.

IEP adjustment

Anytime, you can make modifications to your son's individual education plan (IEP). For a revision meeting, name. Your son may be capable of have an aide go for holiday at the bus. Ask for recommendations, preserve meeting until the organization comes up with a solution.

Adaptation

You need to make a plan for model in the intervening time. Maybe your son might be inclined to take the bus as quickly as in line with week. His self notion will increase with every successful journey. Keep consisting of bus trips in your weekly time desk. It might take some time, but it's miles viable to make the transition depending at the bullying state of affairs.

Weighing the dangers

You can also decide that giving your toddler a revel in to high school every day is well genuinely worth it to make sure his emotional and bodily well-being. While it may appear inconvenient, weigh the professionals and cons to determine what is best in your son in this case.

Parenting a little one with Asperger's Syndrome can be tough. You instinctively want to protect your little one in every state of affairs and it is frequently appropriate. Bullying need to no longer be not noted.

Is it proper to maintain our son off college for a yr?

27. My son attends a private school. He is at grade 4 academically. To seize up socially, we decided to preserve him in Grade 3 for each distinctive 12 months. Your opinion?

School administrators frequently propose that children with Asperger's Syndrome repeat grade levels. Although Asperger's kids are clever, many may be socially immature and feature problems with teachers. Social immaturity is the maximum commonplace purpose for repeating a grade. This concept can frequently do greater damage than unique. Here are a few mind approximately repeating grades before you make a decision to keep your son in 0.33 grade.

Academic boredom

What will the effect of repeating zero.33 grade on a toddler able to instructional excellence? He may be bored, on the way to boom the risk of him having behavioral issues in magnificence.

Continued social adulthood

How can a toddler develop socially mature if he is surrounded thru kids more younger than him? While this corporation is probably greater socially well ideal, it will now not decorate his social adulthood. Asperger's kids may be troubled with the aid of a high-quality social deficit. What takes place if the kid remains socially immature even after a college twelve months? Is it ok to preserve him decrease again?

School offerings What social development opportunities will the university provide to foster social adulthood? The baby will not be challenged academically and could percentage his college day with university college students twelve months more youthful. What is the college's plan to feature to the kid's university day to make certain a nice very last outcomes for the child?

It is vital to deal with any signs and symptoms and symptoms of maturity or instructional weak spot that could have an impact on a infant's capacity to be successful as quick as viable. It is feasible to address social immaturity in an alternative manner. Here are some techniques to assist your infant reach grade 4 in case you want to encourage academic growth and social adulthood.

Social abilties agencies can be positioned with the useful resource of the use of contacting your community Autism help employer or network disabilities offerings center. These companies allow for exercise in planned social settings with steerage from a knowledgeable counselor.

Social golf equipment which might be geared in the course of your infant's specific hobby will provide him an opportunity to meet like-minded kids.

Talk on your toddler's college directors about putting in a peermentoring application. A peer friend can help your infant navigate social situations. Students eligible for the peer-mentoring application should be evaluated, need to be the equal grade degree or a bit older, and must have exceptional grades and conduct.

Repetition of grade stages with the intention to boom social maturity isn't a guarantee of tutorial fulfillment. Research has examined that the consequences are far worse than you may think. A little one being held again for additonal than a yr can result in low vanity and behavior problems. This may additionally moreover even boom the chance of a child turning into a juvenile crook or an adult underachieving. This is a difficult choice.

Sex Education and Puberty

28. What should the school do about intercourse schooling and issues because of early puberty?

There is a lot debate approximately sex education for kids in college. Some undergo in mind intercourse schooling should not be customized and need to observe to each little one in a wonderful way. Others revel in that everyone want to gain expertise of clean facts the equal. Many households need to have entire manage over training in their kids in topics associated with puberty and sexual schooling. However, most choose to artwork with the school.

Asperger's Syndrome kids often attain puberty masses in advance than their chronological age. This can bring about problems at domestic similarly to at college. This is why it's miles vital to create a plan on your little one to deal with those issues. If his university is a part, it will make certain that he receives the aid he calls for. All regions of a infant's schooling might be tormented by early-onset puberty. These areas have to be addressed in the little one's person academic plan. The IEP (or Individual Education Plan) is a crook document that makes inns for children with specific desires. The group meeting can encompass particular goals that address intercourse schooling or puberty.

Parents should furthermore be aware of their roles within the plan. It is critical to educate the child basics, ageand gender-appropriate facts, as early as viable. As he matures and learns greater, he is going to now not come to be crushed afterward. Parent and little one have to talk overtly and use repetition to help with huge issues for the duration of puberty. These are some thoughts to assist Asperger's Syndrome children better apprehend and manipulate puberty, sexual modifications, and other troubles.

Behavior change may be counseled if the child goals assist to differentiate appropriate public and private behaviors. These techniques use repetition of critical instructions or skills to teach the kid and are beneficial at home and at faculty.

Personal self-care skills are crucial for everyone. A toddler with terrible hygiene will affect the whole beauty. Parents must educate the kid the importance of taking regular baths and the usage of deodorant, if vital. It is vital that dad and mom take a look at via with imposing those competencies till they may be conduct. Self-care abilities need to take a look at within the home, but can truely be reinforced at university.

Specific sex schooling subjects can be taught at home and at college. Sex training education at college are commonly short-term with masses of records. This can be overwhelming for the kid with Asperger's Syndrome.

The function of the college in a baby's sexual education and early-onset puberty issues is only determined with the resource of the mother and father' plans for his or her little one. This desire is up to the parents and might range from one member of the family to a few other. It is a incredible concept to request a assembly on the aspect of your toddler's unique schooling coordinator to start to create a plan that meets the desires of Asperger's Syndrome.

Chapter 6: Scholarships

29. I'd want to research greater approximately scholarships for Asperger's patients aged 20.

Asperger's Syndrome is now greater commonplace in young adults and young adults than ever. Colleges and universities are really more privy to the specific needs of Asperger's Syndrome students and provide hotels. Many teens with Asperger's Syndrome have many options and amazing futures. There are plenty of grants and scholarships available to assist pay university costs. Many of those are specially designed for character college college students. People with disabilities may be eligible for presents and scholarships. These are the maximum famous styles of economic beneficial useful resource for college.

Federal gives and espresso interest pupil loans are commonly used for university training. Examples are the Pell Grant and the Stafford mortgage. State scholarships are small annual scholarships given to qualifying university students within the u.S.. One instance is a scholarship software funded with the useful resource of way of a state's lottery software program. These packages regularly have high faculty alternatives and character training options.

Local or network scholarships are every now and then to be had for college children attending the local community college. The university alumni group may additionally fund this scholarship.

Specific scholarships funded in a person's reminiscence may be offered to university students with a common interest. For instance, a overdue doctor's family might probable provide a memorial scholarship to a pre-med student.

Government programs, lottery programs, or nearby organizations also can moreover fund technical college presents. Technical faculties offer certificates guides that train unique trades to adults. These applications normally run a 365 days or and are in reality covered by grants and scholarships.

You can communicate to the economic aid department at the college or college wherein your son is fascinated to find out the data of scholarships and offers. Local colleges can also have financial beneficial useful resource departments that will let you with financing your son's education. The Work Investment Act is a government software program that can be accessed via using your son through his nearby profession center. WIA offers cash to assist out of location human beings. Your network disability offerings branch can guide your look for disability particular scholarships and gives, in addition to career counseling and on-the-hobby training/apprenticeships opportunities.

Your network Autism Support Organization can offer facts on college scholarships and offers for adults with Asperger's Syndrome.

Starting at a Public School

30. My toddler is Asperger's and may be coming into 2d grade in a public university for the number one time. He come to be advocated to visit public college so you can gather extra help with particular desires. Before he starts offevolved, what are a few subjects we've to talk to the vital/teachers? Do we need to get him in Occupational Therapy?

Numerous public schools provide high-quality services to children with Asperger's Syndrome. Every student with special desires is entitled to free, suitable public training (FAPE) inside the United States. The university must offer appropriate training offerings as quickly as the child has been evaluated. Parents can request that the university offer the services on the same time due to the fact the college covers the price.

It is vital to be acquainted with FAPE and criminal recommendations regarding unique needs offerings. Schools may not provide to pay for services that they will be now not able to provide. As the children's advocate and identical member of the educational planning group, it's far as lots due to the fact the mother and father to make sure that the proper services are acquired.

Many colleges can provide a big variety of services to kids with Asperger's Syndrome. To speak your son's admission, you could gain out to the maximum critical or particular education department of the college. These are some topics you might want to hold up at this assembly.

Reveal your toddler's evaluation. It is exceptional to have a right letter of analysis out of your infant's clinical health practitioner.

Request verbally and in writing that the school obtains academic tests and evaluations in all areas: highbrow, speech, conduct, social capabilities, physical treatment, and occupational remedy for sensory troubles, further to satisfactory motor competencies.

Provide copies of your formal evaluations and any tests made thru using his present day-day-day university.

Recognize that it takes time to line up those special services. Even even though your infant is recognized with Asperger's, evaluations are important.

Keep in mind that an educational diagnosis can vary from a systematic prognosis. Even despite the fact that your child has a proper Asperger's Diagnosis, the university can also come decrease returned with an educational evaluation that consists of an trade evaluation. As prolonged due to the fact the offerings supplied meet the kid's desires, strive no longer to strain too much approximately those variations.

Asperger's Syndrome kids frequently get hold of Occupational Therapy as a part of their remedy plans. It all is predicated upon on the needs of every infant. Sensory integration treatment, that may be a shape of occupational therapy, can assist with sensory problems like hypersensitive reaction or sensory-searching for behavior.

The suitable recovery processes may be determined with the aid of your infant's assessment.

Boredom and Lack of Focus

31. My son claims he gets bored at faculty and falls asleep in the course of splendor. Could this be because of the fact he isn't focused?

There are many motives why your son is not enthusiastic about university. Sometimes kids actually do now not like faculty. Sometimes, there are real problems and problems that may be solved to increase participation and morale. A infant who's bored does not paintings to his whole capability. Sleeping kids are not effective! Asperger's Syndrome children can be very targeted, but they may be furthermore regularly fantastically clever. Your son can be bored if he isn't being challenged in his every day obligations. A reading disability or auditory processing sickness may moreover seem to purpose a lack of information, but it could be treated. A lack of awareness additionally can be attributable to anxiety. Your son may additionally additionally seem to lack attention if he's having hassle coping with sensory troubles or social elements of university.

Sleep issues are a commonplace hassle for Asperger's Syndrome kids. Sleep issues, together with insomnia or disturbed sleep, could make it tough to do each day sports. Poor sleep should make your son tired. Sleep deprivation can bring about stress, temper swings which may be volatile, or maybe physical infection. Talk in your clinical physician to find out solutions to your son's sleep troubles. He also can be aware a large difference in his temper and academic general performance if he receives an tremendous night time time's sleep.

School troubles ought to have an effect on a infant's entire existence. Problems at school no longer brilliant show on his document card, however may additionally even display in his low shallowness. School troubles get worse anger troubles and despair. There are such masses of factors at play right here that it is tough to realise your son's particular troubles. The simplest manner to recognize the solution in your son's college issues is to analyze.

A sleep diary will display screen sleep conduct. If terrible sleep is exposed, your medical doctor may inspire you to attempt a melatonin complement to beautify sleep fine. Melatonin is a natural hormone supplement you can purchase in fitness meals stores and a few pharmacies. Dosages variety from one person to the following. Your doctor will help you with that. Improvement will start proper now.

Request new reviews and ask especially for intelligence finding out, beauty/trouble information assessments, and possible learning disability locating out, specifically for auditory processing and interest deficit sickness.

Request an IEP meeting to check the brand new reviews and make adjustments on your son's educational plan. Even if the reviews do now not show display screen adjustments, the IEP must be reviewed due to the fact that his plan is failing him to three degree.

Does your son seem like confused, stressful, or depressed? These emotional conditions are not unusual for people with Asperger's Syndrome. Counseling or medicinal pills may be needed to collect balanced feelings.

School struggles may be depressing for a child with Asperger's Syndrome. With your useful resource, your son can discover success in faculty.

Does my Son need a School Assistant?

32. Is it so critical that my toddler has an assistant in college or can he maintain going

for walks on his non-public as he has up to now? The college will not provide an assistant for him due to the fact he walks, writes, feeds himself, and goes to the rest room on his private. These are the reasons they've got given me to disclaim my petition.

Many children with Asperger's Syndrome are capable of feature nicely enough at a few stage in the university day to keep away from the want of an assistant. It is feasible that almost all of youngsters with Asperger's Syndrome do not need an assistant for every day duties. However, a few kids do need this employer and might be in reality misplaced with out it.

Supplying assistants to college college students can be very highly-priced for university districts. The suggestions will appear very strict regarding the necessities for this organisation. The motives your toddler's college has given for denying an assistant are low priced. Nonetheless, there are times whilst a toddler with Asperger's

Syndrome can have excellent trouble navigating the college day by myself. Here are a fewof the drawbacks that kids with Asperger's Syndrome can also face in some unspecified time in the future of a wellknown college day.

Awkward social situations reason anxiety to assemble, making all activities feel uncomfortable. In addition, the close to social interplay can honestly motive physical ache, in addition to emotional misery.

Sensory problems can deliver a child with Asperger's Syndrome to finish disarray. It is hard to navigate crowded college hallways and cafeterias whilst the sounds, smells, and movement are too much to your sensory device.

Bullying is a massive trouble inside the worldwide of Asperger's Syndrome. In spite of strict no-bullying rules in lots of schools, it is believed that over ninety% of students with Asperger's Syndrome revel in bullying. Bullies are sneaky and university body of workers human beings cannot see everything that takes place in the course of the college day.

With that said, your toddler may be taught to avoid positive conditions that are wonderful to reason him problem. He is aware of who the bullies are. He can be taught to avoid the areas wherein the bullies congregate. Teaching your infant coping strategies can help him make it via the college day effectively. While you are at it, teach him to are looking for help at the same time as he needs it. The instructors and aides at faculty are commonly greater than happy to assist a scholar get from point A to issue B with out physical or emotional trauma.

If you are no longer capable of educate your toddler those precious commands, request assist training those rules from the faculty frame of people Request an IEP review meeting to speak about the elements of war. If the workforce see that your toddler's struggles are interfering alongside with his productiveness, the idea of an assistant may also additionally moreover come up again with a greater fantastic response.

Chapter 7: Problem With Writing Skills

33. My son is going into fourth grade, and has a very difficult time collectively along together with his writing capabilities. Third grade was a venture and luckily we had an information trainer. She allowed me to assist with the e-book critiques and specific massive assignments. I want to put together him to do his personal work this yr, alongside together with his acknowledgement, that there can be more paintings expected from him. Please provide hints.

Many kids with Asperger's Syndrome have first-rate problem with writing competencies. The act of writing falls beneath tremendous motor talents, which is usually a prone location. The perception method of writing additionally can be affected. Your son's conflict to recognize social relationships and conversation, as well as his lack of capacity to make bigger mind on his very own, could have an impact on his writing abilties.

While in zero.33 grade, your son had an exceptional instructor. Another trainer may additionally moreover in no manner once more in form her information of his limitations and her willingness to simply accept your involvement. Preparing him to do his very very personal paintings is important. Here are multiple mind that will let you take little one steps towards independence.

Use occupational treatment strategies at domestic, whether or now not or no longer your son gets formal profession remedy at college or now not. You can discover ebook and movement images that take a look at many occupational remedy potential devices for home use. With a touch extra workout at home, your son can be showing off his new, superior handwriting competencies and will in all likelihood examine calming techniques for sensory overload. What a nice bonus!

Every toddler need to research about employer. It is proper to understand about report folders, locker cabinets, and workplace supply bins. However, employer is a lot extra than retaining track of your papers. It is also about seen schedules, 3-minute timers, and each day calendars. It is set cleaning the house, doing the laundry, and however making it for your physician's appointment with time to spare.

Play video video games that require tempo and accuracy. These video video games will provide a lift for your son's concept techniques. He will become a faster logician.

All of these easy standards or thoughts can be used at home for very little coins, but the viable enhancements are big. Do not neglect about to have your son exercise his newfound abilties. A faux e book report makes an brilliant exercising device. Work on writing talents, time control, using written schedules, and at the identical time as it's miles correct enough to ask for help.

Sometimes, extra huge assistance is desired. It is a notable idea to speak together along with your son's new trainer about his areas of weakness. This teacher may additionally have tips and tips that help your baby become more green while running on his personal. For instance, adjusted assignments which may be broken down into smaller, less tough to cope with steps can increase your toddler's chances of achievement.

Trauma and Anxiety at School

34. My infant, a fifteen yr old with Asperger's Syndrome, became assaulted and sexually pressured by means of a few other pupil at college. He advanced extreme anxiety and has not been able to go back to the university surroundings. School refuses to make connection between the attack and son's worry of the educational surroundings. I surely have attempted domestic training and characteristic no longer felt that it have grow to be successful. I revel in that the college's failure to deal with the state of affairs effectively is the motive that my son has superior this immoderate anxiety, and that they need to want to perform a bit

component is crucial to provide him with an education. While on clinical depart for the anxiety, the university threatened us with truancy, which has paralyzed our son even similarly because of the fact he has advanced separation anxiety as properly. What have to you do?

Your toddler's school revel in is one which most parents wish in no way to encounter. It sounds nightmarish and top notch. However, it takes place too frequently. Children with Asperger's Syndrome are susceptible to anxiety after which their truth will become the nightmare through the palms of a bully, or worse. The school's movements, or loss of motion, have compounded the state of affairs. It may be time for due procedure.

What is due approach? Due system is the order of defensive techniques supplied whilst the child's dad and mom do now not accept as true with the university district's observations or actions. The first step is a mediated meeting. The parents meet with the faculty district and a mediator. This person isn't a college district employee. This man or woman permits the 2 occasions obtain an settlement. If that does not paintings, crook employees, who then compare the hassle consistent with the jail recommendations and make a ruling, pay attention the problem. This ruling will encompass the perfect education plan for the kid and is an expert and legally binding ruling.

If you decide that due way is in order, you should be prepared. Here are some recommendations for you:

Documentation collectively with police facts, scientific information, health practitioner or therapist observations, domestic schooling information, and written statements of the activities can be accumulated and used inside the path of mediation or a listening to.

Request a meeting of the IEP group. Provide the documentation to show the university has did now not offer your son with FAPE. Make a right request to exchange colleges, if feasible.

It looks as if your son will in no way enjoy snug in this putting. If no more public college is to be had, request that the college district cover the charge of a nearby private college that is ready to deal with your son's academic dreams. In the following segment, you could skip thru due way with a mediator. Remember to cite your son's trauma collectively with any police reviews of earlier incidents.

If the mediation fails, you'll need to decide whether or no longer or not to push in advance to a due technique hearing. Once you take this step, the method is from your arms. The being attentive to officer or decide will make the very last choice regarding your son's character schooling plan. The officer need to take all past offenses and actions into hobby as he makes the selections for your baby's education.

Is Mainstream School Best?

35. My 14 year vintage son is in mainstream school however has a declaration. Even so,

every day is a war to get him there masses so that a few days I permit him stay at home. I worry that I've made the wrong desire and that he'd be happier in a extra expert faculty as he certainly doesn't appear like getting everywhere alongside collectively together with his studies.

In the United Kingdom, statemented college students are university college students who have legitimate unique training plans. The declaration is much like the IEP within the United States. The declaration includes the statistics of the academic software program. In the US, all students with special schooling wishes are given an IEP. In the United Kingdom, there are degrees of precise education, the statemented and the non-statemented. The non-statemented college college students usually have an awful lot less extreme needs and are given a greater reserved unique goals plan. Statemented college students normally have a documented evaluation and are eligible for centered offerings.

Mainstreaming youngsters with Asperger 's Syndrome is a famous concept. It follows the regulation of the least restrictive environment for FAPE or, Free Appropriate Public Education. However, mainstreaming isn't the answer for each toddler. Some do a whole lot better in the smaller special training lecture rooms or in possibility colleges focusing on unique goals training. The most effective manner to make certain if an educational environment will art work on your infant is to try it. Statemented college college students deserve the right academic setting to in form their dreams.

If you sense your son's instructional plan isn't always operating or that he isn't making development in his studies, there may be some thing you may do approximately it. You can ask for an early evaluation of his statement. Here are the stairs you have to take:

Discuss your troubles with y our little one's trainer and headmaster. Ask for a letter of assist to be sent to your LEA. Having your infant's teacher on board ought to make a difference.

Write a letter on your LEA's director of education asking for an early evaluation. (Statements are reviewed once every 12 months.) Be wonderful to encompass your issues regarding your infant's schooling and your motives for this have a look at.

You can write a letter in your LEA soliciting for new evaluations. This is feasible if you accept as real at the side of your son's unique education necessities have changed for the cause that final assessment. You want to list in case you anticipate his goals have modified, if you assume he dreams extra assist, a different shape of help, or if you assume he wishes a completely unique sort of academic placing. As before, talk your problems collectively at the side of your son's teacher.

You can also write in your LEA and request a exchange of faculty if you are willing to try every other mainstreamed setting. A university change request is invalid whilst requesting a one-of-a-kind form of university putting. Age may be every different detail to preserve in thoughts. Many 14-three hundred and sixty five days-vintage boys resist university. They might alternatively play video video games and sleep. If university is a terrible revel in, the boy will in all likelihood close down with out a few form of terrific have an impact on.

How can my Son Work Faster?

36. His instructors bitch approximately the reality that it takes him longer to complete an undertaking. So how can I help my son art work quicker so he does no longer fall at the back of in his assignments?

Teachers frequently bitch about the slow art work tempo of university students with Asperger's Syndrome. The loss of language abilties plays a element, similarly to the student's physical obstacles because of the shortage of remarkable motor abilities. The scholar's handwriting abilities are probable awkward and clumsy, for that reason slowing him down. Poor organizational abilties interfere with the student's potential to supply well timed assignments. In addition, many children with Asperger's Syndrome are perfectionists bordering on obsessive behaviors. This motives manage issues.

The sluggish tempo problem is frequently addressed within the scholar's education plan. The pupil is offered reduced workload, time beyond regulation for max assignments, studying assistance in the course of sorting out, and occupational treatment carrying events to enhance awesome motor abilities along with handwriting. The first element you may do is to ensure your son has those special lodges in place to help him become a a fulfillment student. Here are some extra thoughts for you.

Organizational competencies are important for independence. Learning time manipulate techniques, concept manner manage, in addition to fundamental organizational talents like maintaining a each day calendar, developing written lists, and the use of one of a type visible aids will assist our son turn out to be extra efficient.

Remember the significance of normal. Your son plays fine even as he has a tough and fast and normal routine. Work to make his domestic time a persevering with, mounted continuation of his college day. It can also additionally additionally appear like an excessive amount of to you, but children with Asperger's Syndrome attain splendid consolation, consequently becoming greater effective, even as the regular is inflexible.

Practice superb motor abilities physical games and handwriting frequently. Practice will help increase his handwriting velocity. With introduced pace, he can end assignments faster. Taking notes sooner or later of splendor turns into much less hard for him.

Take steps to manipulate obsessive behaviors. Unfortunately, those behaviors are common in kids with Asperger's Syndrome. They can take control and motive many issues. Learn and perform conduct amendment strategies for obsessive and/or compulsive troubles.

Complaining instructors can increase your son's anxiety ranges. Since kids with Asperger's Syndrome are possibly to suffer from anxiety, this terrible input is sure to have an impact to your son. Behavior amendment, treatment, or medication may be needed to manage anxiety because of educational stress. Taking steps to deal with your son's weaknesses will beautify the situation. In addition, it might not damage to schedule a meeting to remind your son's complaining instructors about his educational limitations.

Poor School Attendance

37. My fifteen year vintage grandson who has best had a 60% attendance at college this 365 days has been told he can not go again after vacations. What can I do approximately this?

Regular college attendance isn't always great crucial for exquisite development; it is also the law. However, college university college students with Asperger's Syndrome, like your grandson, might also moreover struggle to meet the attendance requirements because of behavioral troubles together with wrong social interactions, sensory issues like being crushed with the aid of the crowds and commotion, emotional distress along with tension and despair, and exclusive more conventional reasons along aspect infection. Throw within the stubborn teen with an thoughts-set and you could see how resultseasily low attendance comes approximately.

Fortunately, there are unique regulations regarding the expulsion of special dreams college students. The appropriate records is, even in case your grandson is expelled from college, he's nevertheless entitled to a unfastened, suitable, public schooling within the least restrained environment to be had. He might not be capable of attend his regular college, however the school district need to hold to observe his man or woman education plan in an change vicinity. It is important which you recognize your rights and which you observe an appropriate steps at a few diploma inside the method.

Since an expulsion is virtually a change of services, the college should treat it as they might any alternate within the student's IEP. They ought to notify the parents in writing.

The college need to carry out an assessment of the student's abilties. Parents ought to be knowledgeable in writing before this takes area and they may be required to permit the assessment.

An IEP meeting want to be held to determine if the reasons for expulsion have been as a result of the scholar's disabilities. The new assessments are used to determine if the student's services have been appropriate on the time of offense. If the IEP organization individuals find out that the offenses have been due to or had been immediately stimulated through manner of the scholar's disabilities, he can not be expelled. If they discover no correlation a number of the offense and the incapacity, the pupil can be expelled, however remains entitled to the training plan in an exchange putting.

It is crucial which you examine the reasons to your grandson's low attendance, no matter the university district's findings. It may be time to explore distinct alternatives for his schooling. A unique desires college or domestic schooling may be a better healthy for him.

Chapter 8: Fitting In And Making Friends

38. My daughter located her first year at Junior High School fairly difficult as she reveals it very tough to 'in form' in with exclusive women her age. How do I help her address 'turning into in' and making pals?

Junior High School can be a tough transition period for masses children. It is a time at the same time as you aren't a touch kid, however you are not but mature enough to address the traumatic conditions of immoderate university and to be taken into consideration all grown up. It is a time at the equal time as you begin to confront the area together together together with your private mind and opinions. It is a time at the equal time as your frame goes via outstanding exchange. It is a time whilst social connections could make or ruin you.

Girls with Asperger's Syndrome want desperately to make those social connections and suit in with their friends. Unfortunately, social conditions are pretty hard. Your girl will want help inside the direction of this hard time in her lifestyles. Here are a few regions that could motive your female to warfare.

Social competencies are crucial for friendships. Your girl will need to apprehend the way to engage in a set of ladies. Her university may be able to offer social skills groups and probable peer mentoring. Making connections in those settings can also help her obtain out on her private. You also can attempt college and community groups and golf equipment for social workout. Encourage her to join companies which is probably focused on some thing her most critical pursuits are. Examples are academic clubs, sports activities, scouting organizations, network volunteers, and church youngsters enterprise. Using her unique interests to exercise social skills will make it much less complicated for her to loosen up and revel in the approach.

Social communication merits a category all its private. Social communication is covered in social talents, of direction. However, we normally have a tendency to miss about all the nonverbal verbal exchange that occurs in social situations. Nonverbal communication is especially complicated for youngsters with Asperger's Syndrome. Social cues, hand and body gestures, personal area suggestions, and facial expressions make up the majority of someone's communication. You can use flash playing cards with images of feelings, gestures, and expressions to educate your woman approximately nonverbal verbal exchange. You can locate them at the Internet or make a few your self. Role-gambling -way verbal exchange w/nonverbal communique is a few different way you can workout those skills.

Basic self-care abilities are tremendously crucial for pre-young adults. Puberty brings on bodily adjustments that require ordinary private hygiene. Clean body, clean hair, easy tooth, and smooth clothes have to be the guideline of thumb. Without those, your lady will never healthful in. Use visual aids to remind her to take care of herself.

Fitting in is so crucial at this age. If your female continues to conflict, watch for symptoms and signs of unusual stress, anxiety, or melancholy. Any of these signs and symptoms can short spiral out of control.

Problems after School Holidays

39. My fourteen year antique son well-knownshows it pretty difficult to get lower once more into the swing of faculty as soon as off for six weeks and going decrease back to new teachers and new school uniform how can I make this phase less hard for him.

The lazy days of summer season pass all too speedy, leaving college children shaking their heads, questioning how the infinite free time of the holiday disappeared. When you factor inside the want for normal and the struggles with transition and change because of Asperger's Syndrome, it is straightforward to look what a problem the summer season excursion may be.

We will be predisposed to slack in plenty of areas at a few stage within the university vacation. We stay up overdue and sleep in, getting our sleep cycles all out of whack. We snack more on goodies and junk ingredients, eating plenty lots less nutritious substances, causing wild power and mood swings. We neglect approximately approximately our each day schedules and absolutely go along with the glide. Then all at once, we slam at the brakes and try and set subjects back so as for the modern school year. Can you see the disaster prepared to show up? Your toddler with Asperger's Syndrome is probably a complete mess. Here are a few tips that may assist as you are making your way again on your everyday agenda.

Try to stay through normal all three hundred and sixty five days lengthy, retaining bedtimes, hygiene, food, and loose time as you do sooner or later of the university one year.

Stick to your normal time table as plenty as viable. Appointments, errands, family chores, and garden art work are examples of scheduled sports.

Teens with Asperger's Syndrome frequently have sleep troubles. Keep a ordinary bedtime most of the time. Make overdue nights a deal with, not the norm. Use supplements like melatonin to assist improve sleep top notch.

Have snack food on unique activities and not an each day incidence. If you commonly take a look at a completely precise weight loss program, try to stay with it.

Continue all medicinal drugs and dietary supplements. Many human beings see the summer time spoil as a time to slack up on the drugs to store money. Most scientific docs will urge you to preserve the medicines to preserve that stability the drug treatments offer.

Use seen aids each time possible to help your son see the massive photo. Picture schedules, calendar pages, and written lists are some examples of visible aids.

Transition again to highschool uniforms slowly, including shorts and tee shirts in the uniform colors for your son's dresser. Eventually replace every object with actual faculty uniforms.

Check with our university's unique education branch or the college primary to study the identity of your son's new teachers, if the least bit possible. This easy act can assist preserve his tension at bay. Chances are he will recognize photos in remaining three hundred and sixty 5 days's yearbook or at the college internet web page. He can be acquainted with the academics' lecture rooms. These pointers allow you to have an interesting summer time smash and a easy transition once more to highschool inside the fall.

Home Schooling

40. I become questioning what your views are on Home Schooling youngsters with Asperger's?

Many youngsters with Asperger's Syndrome are successfully home schooled. Home education is a developing possibility for households who are uncomfortable with the belief of sending their youngsters off to be encouraged by means of manner of a school room entire of 25-30 of their identical-age friends. Parents are getting to know that domestic training is an opportunity for children with specific wishes and may be the higher choice regularly.

Now that domestic training has a rather big following, locating curriculum picks to wholesome loads of personalities and getting to know styles is as clean as a Google are searching for. Nearly each therapy provided in faculties is available as domestic programs. Speech therapy, neurodevelopmental therapy, imaginative and prescient treatment, bodily remedy, behavioral treatment, and occupational treatment are the maximum not unusual. Most mother and father are capable of reading the strategies from the diverse books and video programs in the market. Many authors do schooling periods, conventions, or even personal counseling thru e-mail or echat.

Home education isn't always for each circle of relatives. It takes pretty some art work and planning on the dad and mom' element and an entire lot of subject and desire on the kid's element. If the parents or the child have troubles with motivation, strength of will, and perseverance, home schooling may be hard. Both dad and mom need to agree that domestic training is the solution and determine to training the child. If you decide to domestic university your child with Asperger's Syndrome, you may want to bear in mind the following factors.

Home training is jail in most international locations. However, the criminal suggestions vary extensively. It is critical that you observe the felony suggestions in your area and follow them. Delight directed learning lends flawlessly to the best hobbies held by using manner of

Chapter 9: Autism Stages

The former categorization device can also moreover have seemed a bit extra easy, but there was pretty a few functionality for ambiguity and interpretation due to the minute variations that frequently separated one from the alternative In order to cope with this, ASD is now divided into 3 tiers, every of which shows the capacity degree of help a affected person can also need.

Level 1 of the ASD The lowest magnificence in the in the meantime is ASD. People at this level will need a few help with troubles collectively with restrained social contact and a loss of planning and organizing talents.

ASD Level 2 - Level 2 is the middle diploma of ASD. At this degree, humans need pretty a few assist and have problems which might be extra seen to outsiders. These problems would possibly embody verbal communique troubles, very slim hobbies, and recurrent, repetitive actions.

ASD Level three - At the severest stop of the spectrum, Level three desires quite a few assist. Level 1 and Level 2 symptoms are however there, but they may be plenty more severe and encompass greater problems. People at this degree ought to have prone social skills and communique skills.

ADULTS WITH AUTISM

Autism is described with the resource of signs and symptoms that impair terrific of existence and typical performance in areas like task and faculty, which encompass problem talking and connecting with others, repetitive conduct, and a confined form of pastimes. Nobody with autism has the same signs and signs and symptoms and signs exactly again. ASD is classed as a spectrum illness because of the large kind of its caution symptoms and symptoms and symptoms and signs, further to the severa consequences and assist necessities that people can also come across.

Without the proper remedies and help, some autistic dad and mom enlarge symptoms and signs that might make everyday living difficult. Some people who want plenty a good deal much less care (additionally known as "high-functioning" people) can also moreover moreover virtually experience "certainly one of a type" from others. They may moreover additionally have had that feeling thinking about the truth that they have been more younger, however they've now not been capable of discover the reason for it.

Similarly, people might not be privy to how they experience or act in a completely unique manner, but others round them need to capture them acting or behaving in every different way. Even despite the fact that autism is most usually recognized in kids, autistic adults might possibly stay unidentified.

Adults who have autistic signs and symptoms but need a lot much less help. The majority of the time, ASD is recognized in more youthful children who are round infant age.

If you are an person who hasn't obtained an autism assessment however thinks you may be on the spectrum, you may be seen as having autism however want a notable deal much much less assist. This turn out to be previously referred to as "immoderate-functioning" autism.

The following are signs and symptoms of person autism:

Social interplay techniques

You have a tough time decoding social signs and symptoms and symptoms and signs and signs and symptoms.

Conversation participation is difficult.

You locate it hard to understand the emotions or mind of others.

You have trouble deciphering humans's face feelings and body language. (It's feasible that you cannot determine whether or not or not or not someone is glad or upset with you.)

You talk in a robotic, monotonous, or flat manner that fails to supply your emotions.

You create your very very own evocative expressions.

It might be hard to recognize rhetorical gadgets like "The early chicken receives the bug" or "Don't appearance a gift horse in the mouth."

When speaking with a person, you decide upon no longer to stare into their eyes.

Whether you are speaking at domestic, with buddies, or at artwork, your speech styles and tonality are the same.

You frequently communicate one or favored topics.

In locations wherein silence is expected, you produce noise.

It's hard to set up and preserve intimate connections.

Restrictive and ordinary actions

You war to govern your emotions and the manner you react to them.

Strong emotions that might bring about meltdowns or outbursts are brought on thru modifications in behavior and expectations.

You have an emotional breakdown in reaction to an sudden event.

When your house are relocated or reorganized, you get sad.

You have strict each day schedules, sporting events, and patterns that must constantly be observed.

You interact in exercising workouts and repeated actions.

Additional caution signs

You have exquisite expertise and ardour for a few unique problem areas (like a historic length, ebook series, movie, enterprise, interest, or discipline of examine).

In one or difficult instructional task areas, you excel appreciably. Certain autistic individuals have to excel in some regions on the equal time as suffering drastically in others.

You are significantly greater or lots an awful lot much less touchy than other humans to sensory enter (which include ache, sound, touch, or perfume).

You consider which you lack coordination or are clumsy.

You like strolling and having amusing on my own greater than with others.

You're seen via manner of others as quirky or scholarly.

You have the ability to investigate complex data and hold them for a long term.

You studies wonderful by means of the use of searching or listening.

Diagnosis of adult autism

There are presently no diagnostic standards for adults with ASD. However, the DSM-5 standards as they stand may be changed and used to this age range.

Adults with ASD are regularly identified thru way of clinicians after a chain of in-individual observations and interactions. They moreover don't forget any signs and symptoms the problem claims to be experiencing.

Bringing up troubles

Any problems you may have with verbal exchange, feelings, behavioral styles, a big form of pastimes, and one among a type subjects can be referred to with you through manner of the clinician.

You'll be requested questions about your upbringing, and your therapist must want to meet collectively with your parents or one-of-a-kind seasoned own family humans in case you need to apprehend your ingrained behavioral patterns.

Your health practitioner also can ask your parents questions from that list, counting on their recollections of you as a kid for in addition statistics, if the diagnostic requirements for children have end up used as a point of reference.

Possible motives

If your health practitioner reveals which you did no longer display off ASD symptoms as a toddler however as an opportunity started displaying them as an adult or adolescent, you could be examined for further highbrow fitness or affective issues. Finding a healthcare agency who will diagnose people with autism may be hard due to the reality the majority of diagnoses are made in kids.

Does individual autism have a take a look at?

No of your age, there are not any clinical finding out for ASD. This manner that strategies like blood trying out or imaging assessments can't be used to perceive ASD. Instead, a scientific doctor will have a examine behaviors to determine whether or no longer a affected person has ASD. Adults often have to cross in man or woman for this, all through which the health practitioner will ask you questions and check out your responses. Self-referred to signs and symptoms and signs and signs and signs also can be taken below attention.

When comparing adults, many psychologists use the Autism Diagnostic Observation Schedule, Second Edition (ADOS-2), a diagnostic check.

Adult self-evaluation ASD questionnaires are available online. These tests embody the Autism Spectrum Quotient (AQ) and its offshoots, which incorporates the AQ-10, AQ-20, and AQ-S. These checks should no longer be taken as being conclusive considering they may be no longer equivalent to a expert evaluation.

Chapter 10: Possibilities Of Getting An Autistic Evaluation

Being identified with ASD as an individual may motive a higher information of who you are and the way you've got interaction with the surroundings. Additionally, it can educate you a manner to decorate affected regions of your existence and paintings higher along with your strengths.

Receiving a analysis may additionally additionally provide you new notion into your early years. Additionally, it would make others close to you extra expertise of and sympathetic in the direction of your wonderful dispositions.

Finding new and modern techniques to use your abilities and abilties can be made less difficult with a more consciousness of your non-public feature. You may moreover are seeking out out assistance that is probably suitable for you in collaboration at the side of your scientific medical doctor and loved ones.

Autism aid for adults

Adults often do now not get the equal degree of assist as kids with ASD. With adults with ASD, cognitive, linguistic, and finished behavioral remedy may additionally moreover occasionally be used as a remedy.

Be conscious that excessive high-quality remedies, such carried out conduct evaluation (ABA), are arguable among autistic groups. Some advocacy corporations, similar to the Autistic Self-Advocacy Network, oppose using ABA.

In elegant, relying on the effects you are having, you have to search for precise assist. This could in all likelihood encompass tension, social isolation, marital issues, or professional challenges. Several options embody:

A psychiatrist or psychologist is able to provide an expert medical assessment of ASD thinking about the reality that they'll be every certified scientific experts. Some psychiatrists even consciousness especially on ASD. These diagnoses additionally may be made through licensed psychologists with a PhD, who also can be less steeply-priced in sure regions.

Official ASD opinions also can be supplied in best jurisdictions through different certified intellectual fitness practitioners, together with social employees. For your health insurance organisation to pay for associated costs like treatment, a right diagnosis can be important. It could also be effective as a way to be eligible for a few country-precise government advantages and duties.

Medicine: You can also take transport of medicine via the use of manner of a psychiatrist. This can reduce the signs and symptoms of conditions like tension or melancholy, that may every so often coexist with ASD.

Social Workers: Supporting someone with autism may be a primary obligation for social human beings. They can be knowledgeable approximately community services and self-assist agencies. Some social human beings might also additionally serve as case managers, assisting within the facilitation of suitable scientific and intellectual fitness treatment.

Adults with autism can also benefit from some of therapeutic modalities, collectively with cognitive behavioral remedy (CBT), physical remedy, and occupational remedy.

An man or woman or enterprise surroundings may be used for giant counseling or treatment furnished by using the use of a psychologist.

Vocational rehabilitation: A counselor for vocational rehabilitation (VR) might also help in assessing your specific working abilities and necessities. They can then help you get a venture or preserve one you already have. Each kingdom has a distinctive version of this governmental service.

Support agency: Many autistic humans have associated with different adults on the autism spectrum in man or woman in addition to via on-line forums and businesses.

If you've got were given been given an ASD analysis, you'll be capable of get help to beautify your terrific of lifestyles and attitude going beforehand. Although adults are an lousy lot tons much less probable than youngsters to get an ASD analysis, extra human beings are requesting to have their autistic signs investigated.

It's viable that receiving a analysis will assist you to get proper of entry to assets, apprehend your very own abilities, and form relationships with different autistic individuals.

CAN PEOPLE WITH AUTISM FALL IN LOVE?

People with autism can also moreover moreover have passionate, lengthy-lasting relationships. People with autism often get into dedicated relationships and/or pick out to be married. However, it's miles a common query that issues some those who are beginning to keep in mind if they may be autistic.

The situation that individuals with autism should battle to fall in love or keep an extended-term courting is regularly primarily based on the subsequent elements: empathy troubles, social issues, rigid idea patterns and sports, and verbal exchange issues.

While all varieties of autism can be tormented by these issues, the point of interest of this talk is on Level 1 or excessive-functioning autism (individuals who may have previously been given an Asperger's syndrome analysis). People with better ranges of autism may be more tormented by special events.

Empathy problems

One of the maximum important misconceptions regarding autistic human beings is that they'll be incapable of feeling empathy. In fact, cognitive empathy is the pleasant kind of empathy that autistic human beings regularly undergo with. Cognitive empathy is making an attempt to recognize what some different man or woman is experiencing based totally totally on their body language and different modes of conversation, further to looking for to assume how you may revel in in that man or woman's shoes.

In evaluation, whilst we revel in affective empathy, we "revel in with" the opportunity character. There is a strong emotional response and feeling of connection. Imagine being with a loved one who is sobbing and notably unhappy. You may also be conscious that you're turning into quite agitated. Or you'll be so suffering from an animal's circumstance that you feel as although you can relate to their struggling. These are examples of emotional empathy, and people with autism are often crushed via manner of the breadth in their stories, a long way from lacking in it. Therefore, those who've autism may additionally furthermore empathically be part of on a deep diploma with others.

Social troubles

Social engagement is frequently tough for human beings with autism. Regardless of the severity of their autism, they nearly honestly conflict to interpret social signs and different human beings, in addition to linguistic subtext. In addition, they frequently go through social stress and fatigue and can need to spend time by myself; all of those elements may moreover make it hard for them to meet humans, date, and installation dedicated relationships.

But it won't recommend you can't have a near connection with someone you care approximately, even though you could discover it tough to address multiple individual right away. In reality, in the route of the early degrees of a relationship, humans with autism often come to be very centered on—even, at instances, obsessed with—a few different individual. For girls with autism, this severe interest on distinct human beings is regularly one of the "unique hobbies" that is a signal of autism. And notwithstanding the reality that many people with autism find out it tough to control large gatherings of humans, they often unique a choice for one or robust connections and pretty understand them.

Restrictive thinking and carrying sports

However, whilst a person with autism does find out the individual they want to spend their lifestyles with, they may find it hard to maintain a dating, and their partner may moreover discover it hard to meet some of their demands.

Autism sufferers regularly enjoy strongly related to nice behaviors and techniques of wondering, making it difficult for them to compromise or adjust their behavior. Close relationships from time to time include compromise, it definitely is difficult for every aspects whilst one associate has autism.

Autism patients frequently battle to particular their emotional needs, which can be difficult in intimate relationships. They want to have trouble expressing their preliminary interest in a person, their needs in a courting, or their emotions for a person else.

Chapter 11: The Right Person Can Be Found

Most people discover relationships to be hard. They may additionally moreover grow to be substantially greater hard when autism is blanketed.

However, plenty of the relationship issues my customers deal with can be resolved with better data and communication on each aspects. A associate may be better capable of recognise your requirements after studying about your autism. You may additionally develop communique techniques that seem greater solid and less hard to deal with.

It is not easy. However, for those autistic people who pick to be in a giant courting—no longer all of them do or need to—they definitely own the potential for every love and love in move lower back.

What to Know Before Beginning a Relationship with a Person with Autism.

There are many tremendous blessings to courting an autistic person, but there also can be a touch gaining knowledge of curve. There are severa myths regarding autism, with a number of the more common that specialize in autistic people and sexual relationships.

Some people think that people with autism are not interested by or incapable of romantic love. But this could no longer be further from the reality.

In reality, companions with autism may be first rate. There are numerous blessings to relationship an autistic person which is probably seldom referred to, albeit you could want to be patient while teaching social symptoms and conventions on your associate.

Can someone with autism date?

Yes! Many autistic parents are extra than capable of dating, having bodily intimacy, and empathizing with their relationships, albeit now not always all autistic human beings.

When it involves relationship, autistic people frequently encounter a unique set of problems, but that does not advise they can not have satisfied, enjoyable relationships.

Dating fulfillment and revel in

According to a 2016 research, the amazing majority (seventy 3%) of high functioning autistic respondents had experienced romantic relationships. In fact, simply 7% of interviewees stated they had no interest in relationship. The studies additionally located that autistic couples cautioned extra dating pleasure than autistic-neurotypical couples.

Similar to this, a 2017 research found that most autistic people (seventy 4%) are content material in their relationships, irrespective of who they'll be relationship. Only nine% of participants said they have been sad with their relationship. 29% of the autistic singles polled expressed remorse approximately their single fame.

Autistic people are much more likely to be single than neurotypical people, regardless of the reality that studies has generally refuted the idea that they may be a whole lot less possibly to be interested in romantic relationships.

For instance, examine from 2017 indicated that simply 50% of humans who've been autistic were in partnerships, in comparison to 70% of folks who had been neurotypical.

A 2019 research additionally verified that relationships with autistic parents regularly terminate quicker. In evaluation to neurotypical people, they fear extra about their future relationships, mainly a way to satisfy capacity love companions, however the reality that that is unimportant. Numerous prolonged-lasting, a hit partnerships with autistic parents have additionally been documented through studies.

BENEFITS OF DATING A PERSON WITH AUTISM.

According to a 2016 research, just 20% of people stated dating an autistic person, indicating that autistic ladies and men extra frequently than not date neurotypical people.

There are severa benefits to being in a courting with someone who is autism, despite the fact that neurotypical individuals may additionally furthermore want to change on the same time as courting an autistic man or woman.

These advantages might probable encompass:

Honesty: It's widely known that autistic people are rather honest. Although it would occasionally appear a touch "brutal," this degree of honesty offers advantages. Knowing that your associate is being actual with you and pronouncing what they mean, mainly at the same time as they may be complimenting you, may additionally additionally increase your revel in of self perception. If you're aware about relationship individuals who generally tend to downplay their ideals or pull away from disagreement, this may be a welcome change of pace.

A courting with an autistic person may additionally additionally appear pretty steady and robust on the grounds that they revel in regularity and order. You could have fewer shocks and additional regularity to your life.

Loyalty: If you are looking for for an extended-term partner, you can get alongside properly with someone who has autism. According to a 2010 research, autistic individuals are frequently an prolonged manner more interested in prolonged-term relationships than they're in brief-term hookups. With the recognition of dating apps and the hookup way of existence, autism can be a welcome alternate of tempo for friendship.

Things to bear in mind

Every dating has its very own particular set of problems that frequently need some model. When courting an autistic man or woman, the equal holds real. Although each individual is precise, there are sure commonplace problems that upward push up even as courting an autistic character.

Autism frequently manifests as trouble interpreting social dynamics and signals, together with:

Sarcastic frame language and tone

flirtingeye-rolling

Statements which is probably detrimental in nature

When dating an autistic man or woman, it is normally critical to be as uncomplicated as you could to save you misunderstandings. If you are outraged or irritated via a few detail your spouse said, it may be greatest to specific how what they did damage you as precisely as you can in preference to assuming they can recognize you are disappointed and why.

Additionally, you may need to be a piece greater direct than conventional on the equal time as expressing your love hobby on the start of the relationship. Some autistic people have a more difficult hassle decoding social indicators, which incorporates whether or not or not or no longer it's miles suitable to lean in for a kiss or ask a person out on a date.

Chapter 12: Adhering To Societal Necessities

Similar to this, know-how social norms and conventions in masses of contexts might be difficult for a person with autism. If your companion couldn't automatically recognize the manner to behave on a date or on the identical time as meeting your buddies and circle of relatives for the primary time, you can possibly want to be data. It could now not suggest that they can not pick out up the ones traditions. Just a bit more direct schooling is needed than for a neurotypical character. That's OK too.

Additionally, a few autistic humans don't forget that "protective"—the workout of concealing one's autism—is needed of them. Although there may be not some factor wrong with searching out to have a look at extra about social alerts and traditions, it's far super to avoid urging your autistic associate to act in every different manner even as you recall that protecting may additionally additionally additionally have some awful repercussions as well (i.E., forcing them to masks). Be as know-how and accepting of them as you can.

Getting overstimulated

Being without issues overstimulated is some distinctive defining trait of autism. Feeling overstimulated in huge social gatherings or sensitive to physical contact are examples of this.

Respecting your companion's limits whilst having sexual or bodily touch is important. In reality, you have to adhere to this advice irrespective of your romantic dating.

A dislike of exchange

Last however now not least, humans with autism frequently warfare to regulate to alternate. It may additionally need a piece extra steerage and lots much less spontaneity than you are aware about so as to have a successful connection with a person who has autism. Your partner may be acquainted with doing such things as consuming the identical element every day, going to bed on the equal time each night time time, and setting their matters away inside the equal area each day.

Your accomplice may additionally want to experience a touch overburdened in case you wonder them with social gatherings. Your spouse can be capable of emotionally prepare for modifications in their agenda or day by day recurring with a few in advance making plans and enough caution. To make the ones gatherings appear like a ordinary part of your accomplice's week, it may additionally be beneficial to designate positive evenings of the week as "social nights."

How to barter your reference to an autistic individual the use of those pointers.

Even notwithstanding the truth that each dating is precise, the following recommendation can be beneficial, mainly in the beginning, as you negotiate your relationship with an autistic character:

When talking, try to be as sincere as you could.

Whenever your partner requests it, supply them region (especially once they have been overstimulated).

If your partner has to take a vacation from socializing, be sympathetic to their wishes.

Find out right away whether or not or not there are any particular strategies that your associate dislikes to be touched (and take a look at in regularly approximately this).

Avoid unexpected your accomplice with an excessive amount of change .

Be conscious that you can locate positive duties less complicated to do than your partner, and make changes as important (e.G., family chore break up).

Be thoughtful of your companion's likely need for regularity and shape.

In conclusion, studies has confirmed that neurotypical and autistic people have a comparable desire in romantic relationships. Simply said, they frequently find it a bit more difficult to understand social signs and symptoms and deal with dating, in particular early in a courting.

The approach of coming across what a associate needs to experience cushty and satisfied in a courting isn't any fantastic from relationship a neurotypical individual, no matter the fact that you may want to make sure versions at the same time as speakme or attractive with an autistic man or woman. Beginnings typically encompass a reading curve.

And all and sundry you date has every benefits and disadvantages. For instance, autistic people frequently show off those functions mainly, which is probably some of the maximum important features for a dedicated partnership. Simply talk in a directed way than you are used to, and be prepared to offer your associate location in the event that they get overstimulated.

In other terms, autistic human beings can and do revel in love and romantic relationships. It can certainly appear a bit precise than how you're acquainted with it to be in a dating with an autistic man or woman.

SUGGESTIONS FOR GETTING ALONG WITH SOMEONE WHO HAS AUTISM

Encourage the autistic character to pay attention to your brow or nostril if preserving eye contact is hard for them.

Open-ended queries are appropriate, along with "What are your plans for the weekend?"

On a date, offer to pay on your date's drink.

Allow your capacity spouse to approach you at the same time as they are prepared.

Find mutual pastimes by way of way of beginning a informal communicate.

As a place to begin for a date pastime, maintain in thoughts a shared interest.

Exchanging contact records

Check to appearance in case you both want to go on extra dates.

Discover the results of autism spectrum illness (ASD) on your dating via using reading greater about it.

Recognize and communicate your partner's sensory needs and troubles.

Find strategies to loosen up, whether or not you do it collectively or privately.

If you want dating steering or assist, are seeking it out from a professional. Several participants in "Love on the Spectrum" have consulted courting counselor Jodi Rodgers for steering.

What Are the Advantages of Dating an Autism Person?

The following trends that make human beings with autism awesome for dating and relationships encompass:

Being capable of express themselves definitely, as an instance, how they enjoy approximately courting.

Asking direct questions which incorporates, "Are you satisfied with this date?"

Being extra capable of feeling emotions than those with out ASD.

Having a piece possibility of betraying their courting; being devoted.

Observing minute records approximately their relationship that others might likely overlook.

Knowing their accomplice's options, alongside side a favorite emblem of chocolate bar, and bringing them gives that mirror their possibilities.

Being very facts in their lover and owning a totally herbal coronary heart.

Having the patience to wait patiently for their partner to complete their drink.

Autism in Adults: Variability

Autism in adults is available in numerous paperwork.

Some autistic humans have carried out professions in competitive industries together with statistics era, robotics, and online game development.

Some human beings integrate strolling detail-time with the usage of sunlight hours services and packages.

Some humans stay in protected environments due to the fact they're now not able to art work.

Some humans with autism are contentedly married or in relationships.

Some human beings have romantic relationships.

Some humans battle to construct reciprocal, meaningful connections with their buddies.

It is certainly as difficult to give an explanation for or offer help to adults with autism as it's far to youngsters due to those outstanding variances.

Success in Adults with Autism

Some adults who've been diagnosed with autism pass right away to have a hit lives. Many of them have full-time jobs, and others are thankfully married or in relationships. For more youthful humans at the spectrum who want to manual pleasant, impartial lives, a few have even emerged as feature models. Just some examples of such role models are:

Temple Grandin is an writer, lecturer, and expert in animal husbandry.

Stephen Shore is a lecturer, writer, musician, and public speaker.

Speaker and creator John Elder Robison

Dan Ackroyd is a radio host, actor, and singer.

Actor Daryl Hannah

These people, alongside aspect some others, are vocal supporters of autism. Many autistic humans and their households have interaction in public discourse about their stories and provide information and steering.

Serious Issues

While some autistic people with excessive functioning are a fulfillment, many have remarkable problems. Surprisingly, having "excessive" autism might not regularly offer the largest mission to finding a activity or maybe experiencing private pride.

Because they will "pass" as neurotypical while attempting to cope with immoderate anxiety, sensory disorder, and social/communication difficulties, better functioning folks are every now and then at a larger drawback.

A area to a third of autistic people are non-verbal or minimally verbal from early infancy, because of this they may be unable to utilize spoken language or have immoderate difficulties with it.

Recent studies have tested that people with autism regularly behave extra violently inside the course of others, in particular their caregivers.

Naturally, angry, non-verbal humans with autism are unable to feature in everyday environments or employment. In preferred, parents with autism are sincere and honest; the majority are preoccupied with their pastime and seldom permit social interactions or extracurricular hobbies divert them.

Many humans very own terrific abilities in fields like computer programming, mathematics, music, drawing, making plans, and the visible arts. Even although it is probably challenging for autistic humans to prepare and manage their personal areas and schedules, many become terrific employers and those.

Chapter 13: How Asperger Syndrome Affects Child's Life?

How Asperger Syndrome Looks Like?

As stated above, a baby with Asperger syndrome reveals many traits concerning impairments in socialization, cognition, verbal exchange, and sensation. These impairments vary amongst great children and exist on a continuum beginning from excessive to minor. Coping with individuals with Asperger syndrome may be difficult because of their particular variations. Those who've interplay with the ones kids often locate it hard to conform to the everyday modifications of their behavioral abilities. It might also appear as though the scholar you educate in recent times is a completely special individual from the satisfactory you taught the day before today. Based on thorough studies through manner of experts on Asperger syndrome, the following are not unusual dispositions observed in people with Asperger syndrome:

Social Challenges

Lack of records of social cues

Difficulty deciphering exclusive children's phrases

Challenges assignment reciprocal verbal exchange

Tendency to repetitively talk without impacting the listener

Intense awareness on a unmarried topic of interest.

Communication Challenges

Difficulty facts social nuances collectively with sarcasm or metaphor.

Repetition of the very last phrases without conveying proper because of this

Poor judgment of personal region, together with standing too close to others

Abnormal eye contact behavior

Unrelated facial expressions and gestures

Cognition Challenges

Poor trouble-solving and organizational skills

Obsessive and narrowly described pastimes

Concrete, literal wondering

Difficulties generalizing and utilising positioned statistics and capabilities at some stage in numerous situations, settings, and those.

Sensory and Motor Challenges

Over or below-sensitivity to sure sensory stimuli, including ache

Difficulty with top notch motor activities like writing

Impact of Asperger Syndrome on a Child

Asperger syndrome offers various social and behavioral problems that disrupt a toddler's day by day lifestyles. As mentioned in advance, a little one with Asperger syndrome does not proactively behave otherwise from one-of-a-kind youngsters their age. Instead, their behavior is right away linked to the neurological issues in their thoughts resulting from this situation. The following are a few not unusual demanding situations confronted thru kids with Asperger syndrome in their each day lives:

Socialization

Humans are social animals, and social publicity is essential for a children's boom and improvement proper into a nicely-rounded person. However, children with Asperger syndrome are deprived of the social interplay they require to flourish. Social impairments pose the finest traumatic situations for university university college students with this disorder. Every little one wishes buddies to boom their social competencies inside society, but Asperger syndrome hampers their natural intuition to shape friendships, causing them to revel in disconnected from their buddies. Building and keeping social friendships are specifically hard for children with this ailment because of their problems in know-how social problems, deciphering others' terms, and comprehension problems. Consequently, many college students with Asperger syndrome emerge as targets of bullying, teasing, and victimization via using their friends. The following are common socialization troubles faced through kids with Asperger syndrome:

Conversational style: Individuals with Asperger syndrome often lack conversational talents and interact in a single-sided interactions that may not interest their communication companions or institution. They may additionally deliver the effect of being talked at rather than taking component in reciprocal conversations, which hinders their verbal exchange inside a social context.

Bluntness: Children with Asperger syndrome frequently display off symptoms and symptoms of bluntness and can say subjects that appear impolite and insensitive. They will be inclined to blurt out a few component involves thoughts without thinking about whether or not or now not their statements are suitable for the scenario.

Lack of implementation of social rules: Students with Asperger syndrome war with utilizing social suggestions to specific situations or activities. They might also moreover studies social abilities without truly knowledge while and the way to region into effect them. For example, whilst occasional burping among younger boys may be perfect once they stand up in personal regions on occasion. But a baby laid low with Asperger syndrome doesn't understand the modifications in social setting and he should do repetitive burping inside the center of a class mistakenly perceiving burping to be socially desirable.

Communication

Children with Asperger syndrome generally have proper grammar and vocabulary competencies that, in a few cases, surpass the ones in their generally growing friends. However, they experience deficits in verbal and non-verbal communique. Some not unusual conversation demanding situations faced through those children are as follows:

Social elements of language: Children with Asperger syndrome often showcase splendid language getting to know styles in assessment to their peers. They may additionally engage in first-rate discussions approximately a unmarried subject remember this is of little or no hobby to others. They also can moreover communicate in an exaggerated or monotone style, which could seem tremendous amongst their age institution. These children may moreover show a language-related psychiatric disease called 'Echolalia,' which includes repeating a person else's spoken terms with very little social which means. Children with Asperger syndrome might also war to recognise the common expertise of famous English phrases, which encompass 'I heard it at the grapevine' or 'Elvis has left the building.' These terms deliver one-of-a-type meanings depending at the context in which they will be used, but a infant with Asperger syndrome may additionally interpret them genuinely and no longer recognize their supposed figurative due to this.

Abstract thoughts: Many languages require a particular data of precis requirements like metaphors, parables, phrases, irony, sarcasm, and idioms. These ideas characteristic the essential constructing blocks of language, and comprehending them is critical for proper language acquisition. However, youngsters with Asperger syndrome frequently struggle to realize languages that encompass those summary requirements.

Body language and non-verbal communication: Children with Asperger syndrome find out it difficult to expose suitable frame language and non-verbal conversation in social settings. They also can moreover showcase limited or unrelated facial expressions and gestures, awkward body language, and troubles with social proximity, together with fame too close to or too a ways away throughout conversations internal their social circles. These children moreover face issues in information the facial expressions and frame language of their buddies.

Cognition

Children with Asperger syndrome typically have not unusual to above-commonplace intelligence compared to their buddies of the identical age. They often personal excessive tiers of hobby and might showcase information and pursuits beyond their age degree. However, Asperger syndrome can also purpose cognitive deficits that might pose traumatic situations in instructional sports activities activities. Some common examples of these deficits are as follows:

Academic worrying situations: Despite having ordinary intelligence, youngsters with Asperger syndrome regularly revel in cognitive problems that impact their instructional typical basic overall performance. They might also additionally struggle with trouble-fixing and organizational talents, show concrete literal wondering, and face problems in statistics precis requirements. Additionally, those kids might also additionally moreover grow to be fixated on particular pastimes.

Emotions and pressure: Asperger syndrome is a neurological disorder, and children suffering from it do no longer consciously pick to act the way they regularly do. As a result, when they experience extreme emotions, their choice-making and conduct may also moreover grow to be greater pushed through emotions than common sense. It's as if the thinking center in their mind will become a good deal much less energetic even as the emotional middle will become extra outstanding. In many times, these kids can also react rapidly without thinking about the consequences. Even within the event that they examine greater best behaviors, they will nevertheless show off odd behaviors while underneath pressure and revert to their default aggressive behavior.

Inability to generalize records: Children with Asperger syndrome regularly own robust memorization talents, but they commonly usually tend to shop information as disconnected information of their minds. Despite their right memory, those kids battle to use statistics and employ their information effectively.

Note: It's vital to bear in mind that all of us with Asperger syndrome is particular, and the worrying situations they face can range. These descriptions offer a trendy facts of common issues related to the situation.

.